Student Learning Guic

Karen A. Piotrowski, RNC, MSN
Assistant Professor of Nursing, D'Youville College,
Buffalo, New York

To Accompany

Fifth Edition

MATERNITY & GYNECOLOGIC CARE

The Nurse and the Family

Irene M. Bobak, RN, MS, PhD, FAAN
Professor Emerita, San Francisco State University,
San Francisco, California

Margaret Duncan Jensen, RN, MS
Professor Emeritus, San Jose State University,
San Jose, California

Printed in the United States of America

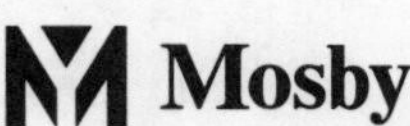

St. Louis Baltimore Boston Chicago London Philadelphia Sydney Toronto

Contents

CHAPTER 1 PERINATAL AND WOMEN'S HEALTH NURSING

1. Describe the health care focus for each of the following nurses:
   - Perinatal nurse – pregnant women
   - Neonatal nurse – newborns
   - Gynecologic nurse – nonpregnant women

2. Give an example of a *Specific* nursing activity that would reflect each of the following perinatal/women's health nursing roles:
   - Caregiver
   - Teacher/educator
   - Advocate
   - Manager
   - Researcher
   - Political activist
   - Change agent

3. Imagine that you are the nursing director of an inner-city prenatal clinic that serves a large number of unmarried teenage women. Describe five nursing services you would provide for these women that would help to reduce the risk of neonatal morbidity, mortality, and low birth weight. Use the statistical data and risk behaviors presented in this chapter to support your proposal.

4. *True or false:* Circle "T" if true or "F" if false for each of the following statements. Correct the false statements.

T F The perinatal period refers to the first 4 weeks of an infant's life.

T F Birthrate refers to the number of births per 1000 women 15 to 44 years of age.

T F The largest increase in the birthrate has been noted among women in their early teens (15 to 17) and women between 35 and 44 years of age.

T F An abortion refers to the expulsion/removal of an embryo/fetus from the uterus at 20 weeks' gestation or less, weighing less than 500 g or measuring 25 cm or less.

T F Perinatal mortality rate refers to the number of stillbirths and infant deaths under 1 year of age per 1000 live births.

T F An increase in births to unmarried women has been noted, especially among white women.

T F A low-birth-weight (LBW) infant is defined as a baby weighing less than 4 lb at birth.

T F The number of low-birth-weight infants can be substantially reduced through perfection of advanced technology.

T F The U.S. ranking of 21st for infant mortality among industrialized nations relates to inadequate prenatal care and socioeconomic barriers for childbearing women.

T F The maternal mortality rate reflects the number of women per 1000 population who die as a result of pregnancy.

5. Nursing diagnoses are used to guide nursing interventions for both the well and the sick client.
   A. Compare and contrast the characteristics of **typical problem nursing diagnoses** with **wellness nursing diagnoses.**
   B. List five nursing diagnoses that you have identified for your low-risk perinatal clients. Evaluate each diagnosis to determine whether it is a typical problem diagnosis or a wellness diagnosis. For those identified as problem diagnoses, determine if they could be converted to wellness diagnoses.

CHAPTER 2 THE FAMILY, A UNIT OF CARE

1. *Matching:* Match the family described in Column I with the appropriate classification in Column II.

COLUMN I	*COLUMN II*
A. Mary and James are a married couple living with their new baby boy, Alex.	____. Binuclear family
B. Alice and John are divorced and share joint custody of their three children.	____. Extended family
C. Jane and Andrew live with their parents, Mr. and Mrs. Smith.	____. Homosexual family
D. Miss Oz lives with her 8-year-old adopted Korean daughter, Kim.	____. Nuclear family of procreation
E. Jacob and Rebeccah are an Amish couple who live on Jacob's family farm with their children.	____. Single parent family
F. Susan and Thomas are married and live with their child, Tim, and Susan's mother, Lisa.	____. Blended, combined, reconstituted family
G. The Pace family consists of Sam, his second wife Jean, and Jean's two sons.	____. Communal family
H. Michael and Tom are a gay couple living with Tom's daughter, Sally.	____. Nuclear family of orientation

2. Describe the conceptual framework of each of the following family theories:
   - Structural-functional theory
   - Developmental theory
   - Interactional theory

3. Choose the cultural concept that most accurately reflects each of the following descriptions.
   A. Mrs. Mendez, a newly delivered Mexican-American woman, tells the nurse not to include certain foods on her meal tray, since her mother told her to avoid those foods while breast-feeding. The nurse tells her that she doesn't have to avoid any foods and should eat whatever she desires.
   B. Mrs. Kim, an immigrant from Vietnam, has lived in the United States for 1 year. She tells you that she enjoys the comfort of wearing blue jeans and sneakers on casual occasions such as shopping, even though she never would have done so in Vietnam.
   C. A family of Cambodian refugees emigrated to the United States and have been living in San Diego for more than 5 years. The parents express concern about their children, ages 10, 13, and 16, stating, "The children act so differently now. They are less respectful to us, want to eat only American food, and go to rock concerts. It's hard to believe they are our children."
   D. The Amish are an important ethnic community, primarily located in Lancaster, Pennsylvania.
   E. The nurse is preparing a healthy diet plan for Mrs. Symanski. In doing so, she takes the time to include the Polish foods that are favorites of Mrs. Symanski.

4. Imagine that you are a nurse working in a prenatal clinic with a client population that is primarily Hispanic. What measures would you use to facilitate culturally sensitive communication between yourself and your clients?

5. Mrs. Reynolds is a 32-year-old primipara who gave birth to a 9-lb 6-oz boy at 42 weeks' gestation, following a long and difficult labor. A cesarean birth was required as a result of cephalopelvic disproportion (CPD) and fetal distress. Her baby is now 6 hours old and was transferred to the neonatal intensive care nursery (NIC) for observation and treatment of hypoglycemia.
   A. Using a crisis intervention framework, discuss how you would assess the crisis potential of this situation.
   B. Describe four specific nursing measures you would use to prevent the occurrence of a crisis.

6. **Family crossword puzzle**

ACROSS:

3. Coping mechanisms that people or families use, which lead to a resolution of a problem.
5. Process in which family integrates members into society.
9. Economic, religious, kinship, and political beliefs and social customs around which the family unit functions.
11. Recognizing that people from different cultural backgrounds actually see the same situations differently reflects the concept of cultural ________.
12. Family group consisting of parents and their dependent children; the traditional American family.
14. The theory that conceives of the family as a unit of interacting personalities, not necessarily bound by legal or contractual agreements, that exists as long as interaction is taking place.
15. One's interpretation of an event, which may be different from another's and may be altered by age, experience, or emotional states.
16. Type of crisis that involves a threat to a person's sense of integrity; birth of a preterm infant, spontaneous abortion.

DOWN:

1. Way in which individuals handle a given situation threatening to their sense of well-being.
2. Determining the allocation of resources and ensuring financial security of family members reflects the ____ function of the family.
4. Composed of two or more people who are emotionally involved with each other and live in close geographic proximity.
6. Process in which one cultural group loses its identity and becomes a part of the dominant culture.
7. Personal belief about worth that acts as a standard to guide one's behavior.
8. Being centered in one's own cultural system, judging the world in general by the standards established in that particular system.
10. Theory in which the person rather than the role is significant and the family process is one of interaction over the life cycle of the family.
13. Crisis that evolves over time and is the result of normal growth and development.

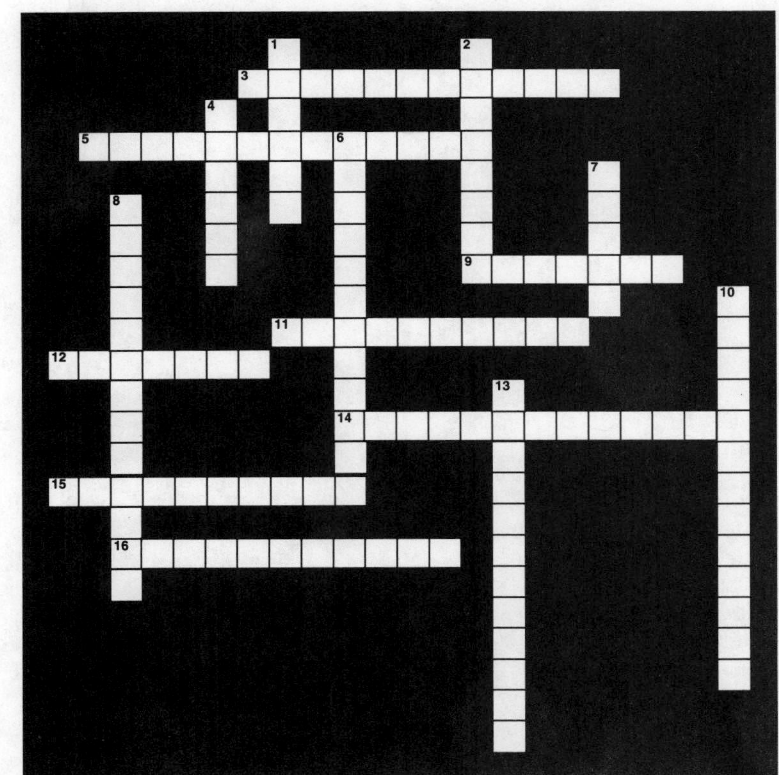

CHAPTER 3 CULTURE AND ETHNICITY

1. You are a nurse caring for Mary Adams, a typical American woman in labor. Describe specific measures you would use to meet Mary's need for territoriality.

2. Touch is often used by nurses when providing physical care and emotional support for clients. Discuss how you would ensure that touch is used in a manner that demonstrates appreciation of your client's cultural preference.

3. How would you determine whether the beliefs and behaviors of a client represent an internal or external locus of control?

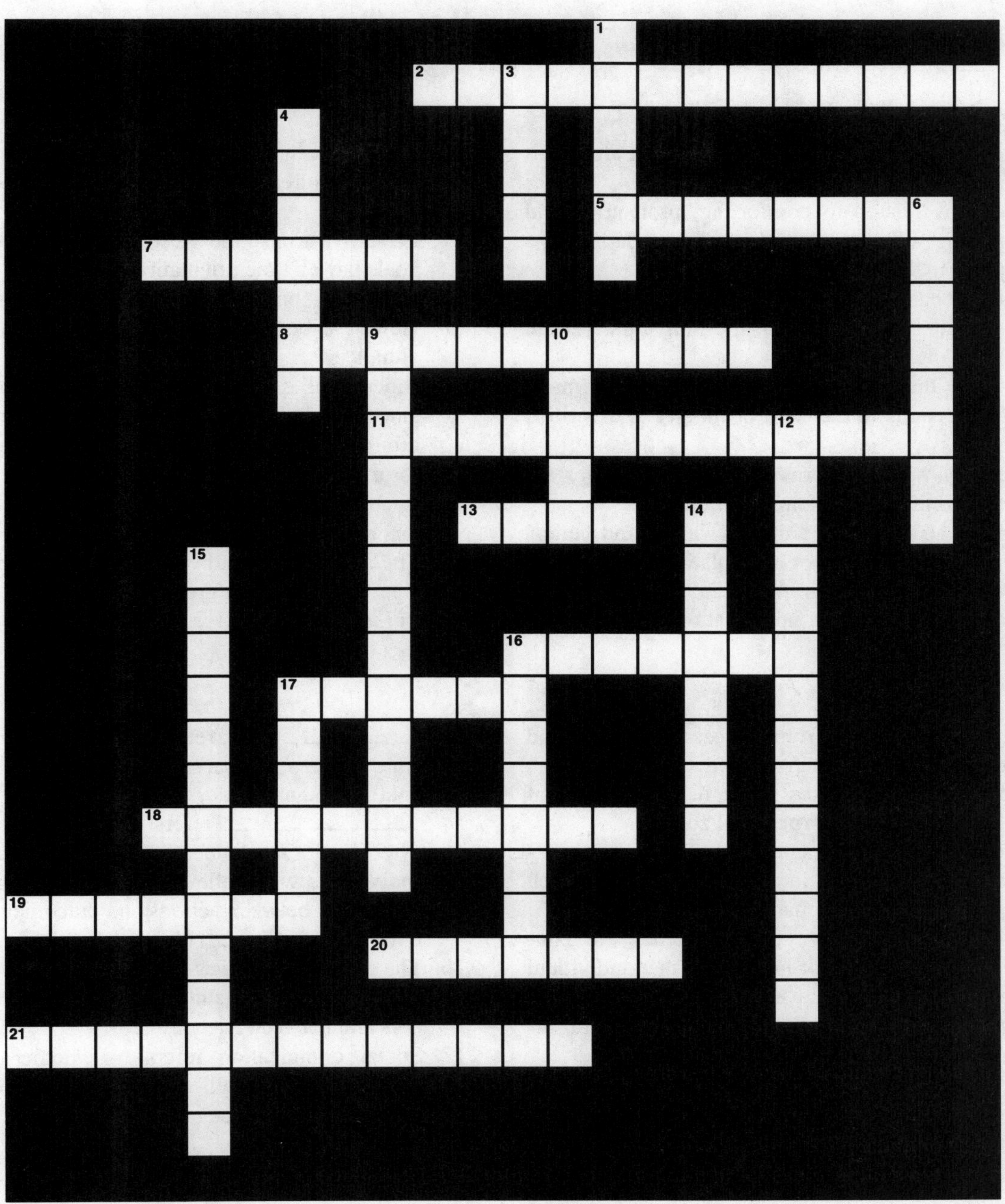

4. **Cultural crossword**

ACROSS:

2. Culturally based health care practices that are harmful to the health status of the individual.
5. Interactions related to comforting, protecting, and lovemaking among persons in close relationships take place in the zone.
7. Culturally based health care practices that have no effect on the health status of the individual yet are integrated into their behavior.
8. A culture that delegates responsibility for many family decisions to the wife or mother is described as ____.
11. Process by which patterns of cultural behavior are modified to fit into the dominant culture.
13. Persons who cling to traditional values and beliefs with little motivation for formulating future goals have a time orientation in the ____.
16. Persons who have little appreciation for the future or the past and who often do not adhere to a strict time-structured schedule have a time orientation in the ____.
17. Persons who use the present to achieve tomorrow's goals have a time orientation in the ____.
18. Culturally based health care practices that are viewed as beneficial to the health status of the individual.
19. Biocultural ____ explores the biologic differences among individuals of various racial and cultural groups as well as the biologic adaptive efforts necessary for homeostasis.
20. A communication variable influenced by such factors as ethnic group and geographic location.
21. The ability of an individual or persons representing a particular cultural group to plan activities that control nature is termed ____ control.

DOWN:

1. The ____ zone ranges from 12 feet and beyond and is outside the sphere of personal involvement.
3. All communication takes place in the context of ____, referred to as interpersonal zones.
4. Organizational structures of the environment that affect and influence the individual and with which there is a continuous exchange of energy.
6. Individuals who believe that outcomes are controlled by fate, chance, or luck rather than individual actions are said to have an ____ locus of control.
9. An approach to nursing that appreciates cultural diversity is ____ nursing.
10. Family ____ are patterns of wants, goals, feelings, attitudes, and actions that family members have for themselves and others in the family.
12. ____________ refers to feelings or attitudes toward an area or space that involve possessiveness, control, and authority.
14. ____________ refers to gestures, stances, and eye behavior used when relating to others.
15. Individuals who believe that a contingent relationship exists between actions and outcomes are said to have an internal ____. (3 words)
16. The ____ zone ranges from 18 inches to 4 feet and is space usually maintained between family members and between friends.
17. Social organization refers to whether a cultural group organizes itself around the ____ unit and the degree of importance it places upon it.

CHAPTER 4 LEGAL AND ETHICAL ISSUES

1. Compare and contrast each of the following methods currently used to define the scope of nursing practice and the minimum requirements for performance of nursing duties:
   - Nurse practice acts
   - Standards of nursing care determined by professional organizations such as the ANA and NAACOG (AWHONN)
   - Agency policy and procedures

2. Imagine you are in charge of a low-risk newborn nursery. How would you establish and implement a process of quality assurance?

3. For each of the situations described below, discuss your legal and ethical responsibility as well as the action you would take.

   A. The physician has just written orders for one of your postpartum clients. The medication order is difficult to read, but you are pretty sure that the order is for methylergonovine maleate (Methergine), 0.4 mg.

   B. Mrs. Andrews has been admitted to your labor and birth unit for an elective abortion. The results of an amniocentesis indicate that the fetus has Down syndrome. You are opposed to elective abortion under any circumstances.

   C. It is 2 AM and you are the primary nurse for Ms. Doe, a woman in active labor. For the past several contractions, when assessing the external monitor strip, you note definite signs of distress in the fetal heart patterns. You notify the physician, who tells you not to worry, and he will check her in the morning.

   D. Mrs. Randell is to have an abdominal hysterectomy with removal of both uterine (fallopian) tubes and ovaries. You bring in the surgical consent for her to sign. She tells you that she is having second thoughts about the surgery and wishes she had asked her physician if there were alternatives.

   E. You are a new graduate nurse from a BSN program. After 1 month working on a busy labor and delivery unit, you are placed in charge for the day because of short staffing. They tell you that you should be able to handle the situation since you have your degree. However, you do not feel ready for such a major responsibility, especially because there are not enough nurses on duty to effectively care for the number of clients.

   F. You are working the night shift in the transition newborn nursery. There are many newborn babies to observe. The nurse you are to work with arrives on the unit impaired by alcohol consumption. You like her and do not want to get her into trouble.

   G. In reviewing your nurse's notes for one of your clients, you notice that you made a charting error.

   H. While caring for two newly delivered mothers in the recovery room, you mistakenly give methylergonovine maleate (Methergine) to the wrong woman.

4. As a professional nurse, it is important to identify whether the nursing activities you perform are independent or dependent.

   A. Describe the difference between independent nursing activities and dependent nursing activities, *and* give an example of each.

   B. List the interventions you performed during one of your clinical experiences. Label each of the interventions as (I) independent or (D) dependent.

5. As part of a quality assurance program, you are assigned to review the nurses' notes on a postpartum unit. Describe the criteria you would use to evaluate the quality of the nurses' notes you review.

6. What are your ethical responsibilities as a student nurse?

CHAPTER 5 NURSING RESEARCH IN MATERNITY AND GYNECOLOGIC CARE

1. Imagine you are a nurse manager of a low-risk postpartum unit. Describe how you would establish a nursing research focus with the nurses on your unit.

2. Research can be conducted using a quantitative or a qualitative approach.
   A. Compare and contrast the characteristics of a quantitative and a qualitative approach to research.
   B. Search the literature for an example of a quantitative research study and a qualitative research study.
   C. Describe the specific differences noted when comparing each study.

3. How would you describe your role as a nursing student with regard to nursing research.

CHAPTER 6 REPRODUCTION AND SEXUALITY

1. A nurse working in the field of women's health must have knowledge of the female and male reproductive systems, including its internal and external structures, the interrelationship of these structures, and their normal characteristics. Label each of the following illustrations as indicated. Then, on a separate sheet of paper, describe the normal characteristics and function of each structure.

   A. **Female genitalia:**

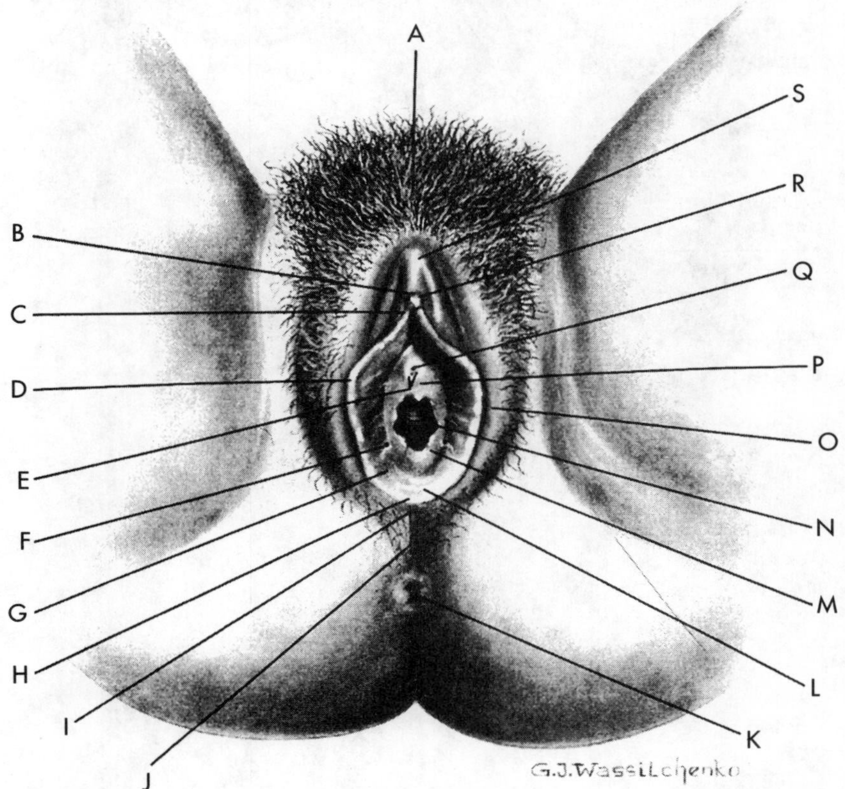

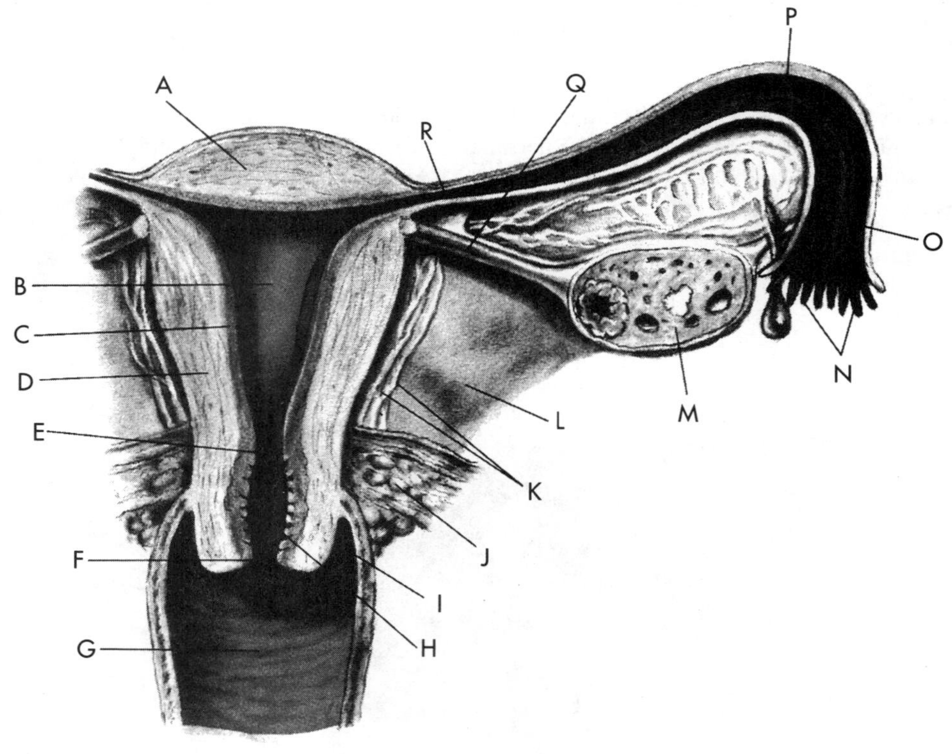

B. **Female breast:**

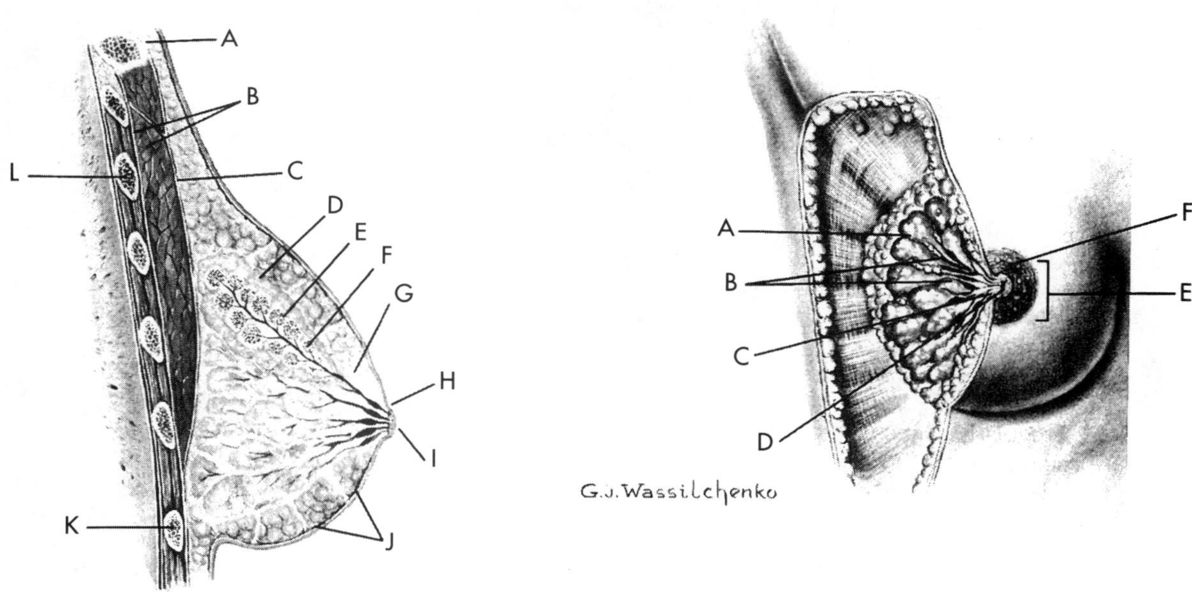

C. **Female pelvis:**

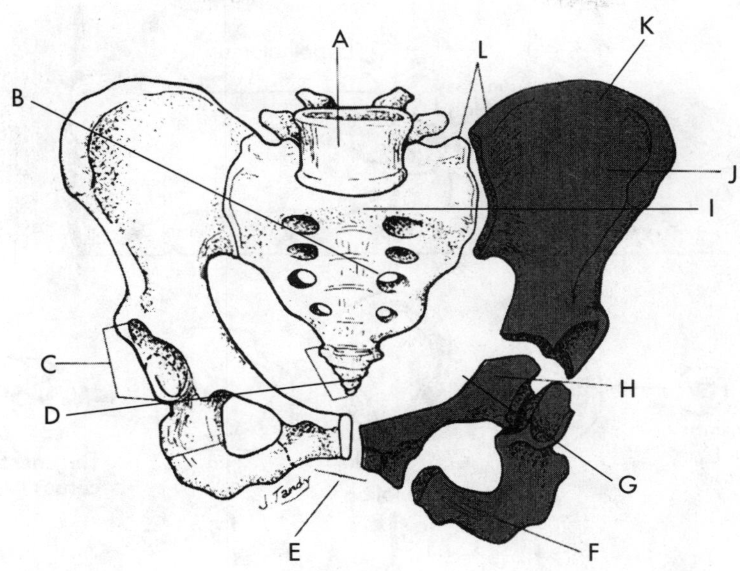

D. **Male genitalia:**

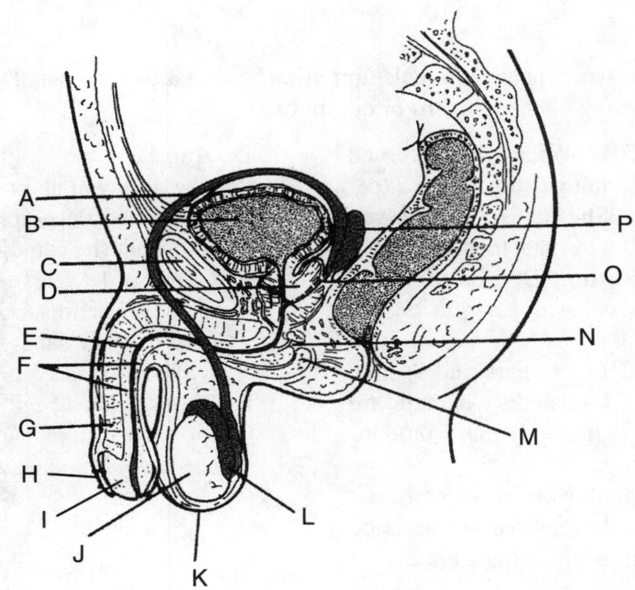

2. The diagram below illustrates the cyclic changes that occur during the menstrual cycle of a woman of childbearing age. Label the diagram as indicated.

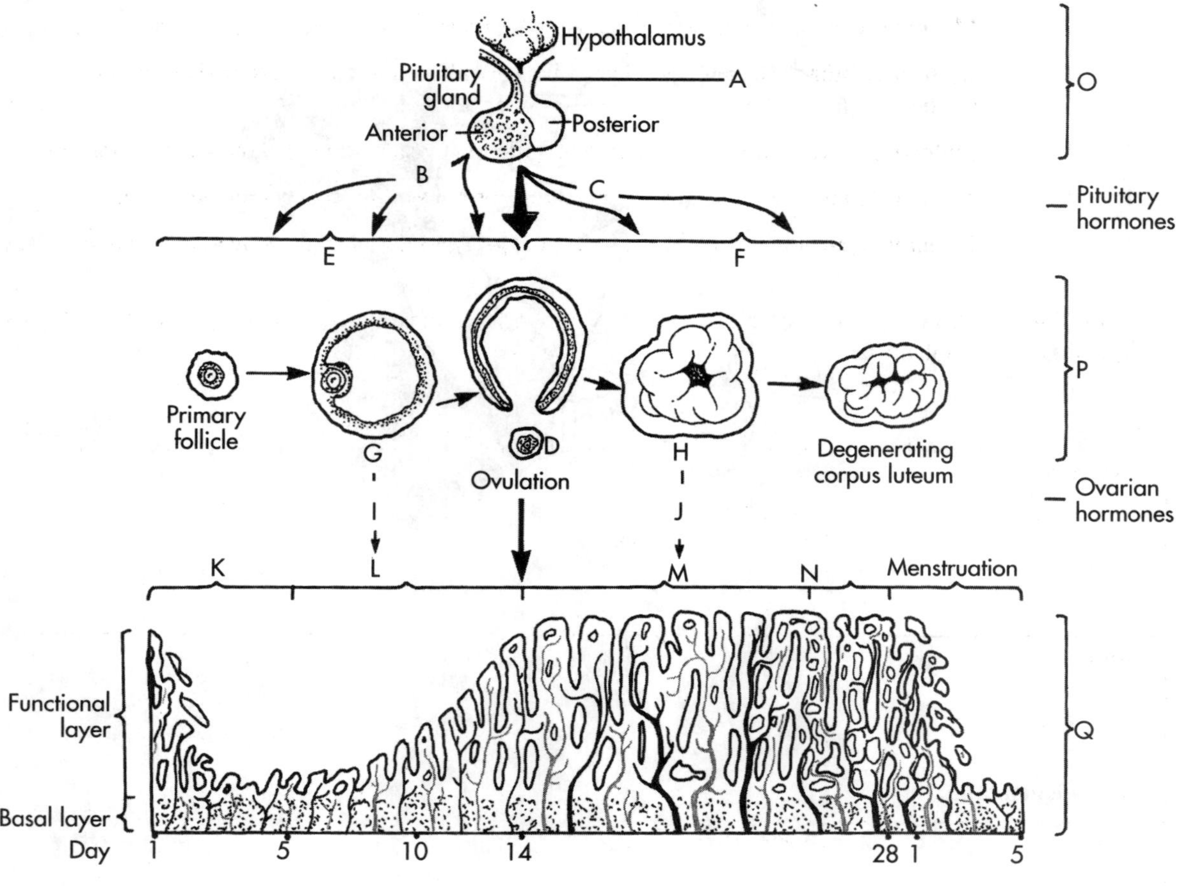

3. Imagine that you are a nurse working at a clinic that provides health care to women. Describe how you would respond to each of the following client concerns or questions.

A. Katherine, a newly married woman, is concerned that she did not bleed during her first coital experience with her husband. She states, "I was a virgin and always thought you had to bleed when you had sex for the first time. Do you think my husband will still believe I was a virgin on our wedding night?"

B. Susan has been married for 5 years and is now trying to get pregnant. She wonders if there are signs she could observe in her body that would indicate that she is ovulating.

C. When teaching a group of women about breast self-examination (BSE), they ask you to describe the normal characteristics of the female breast.

D. Angela is the single parent of a 1-year-old boy. She asks you about what to expect with regard to his sexual development over the next few years and what she can do to foster that development.

E. Gloria is 48 years old and is beginning to experience perimenopausal changes. She expresses concern that her satisfying sex life with her husband will be adversely affected by these changes.

F. Debra has just been diagnosed as being pregnant for the first time. Her rubella titer indicates that she is not immune.

4. *True or false:* Circle "T" if true or "F" if false for each of the following statements. Correct the false statements.

T F The prepregnancy size of a woman's breasts are a major influence on her ability to breast-feed.

T F Breast self-examination (BSE) is best performed 5 days before menstruation.

T F Dysmenorrhea is most often associated with ovulatory cycles.

T F Pregnancy is not possible until at least 1 year of menstrual cycles have occurred following menarche.

T F Variations in the length of the luteal phase account for almost all variations in the length of menstrual cycles.

T F Menopause is dated with certainty once 1 year has passed since the last menstrual period.

T F Both spermatogenesis and sperm are adversely affected by a hot external environment and limitations on the mobility of the testes.

T F Following a vasectomy, there should be little to no ejaculation of semen during orgasm.

T F The development of core gender identity is normally completed during adolescence.

T F Parenting demands can adversely affect the partner relationship and lead to sexual dysfunction.

5. Complete the following table related to the phases of the **human sexual response** as described by Masters and Johnson and Helen Kaplan:

FOUR PHASE	BIPHASIC	MALE RESPONSE	FEMALE RESPONSE
Excitement	Vasocongestive		
Plateau			
Orgasmic	Reflex clonic		
Resolution			

6. *Matching:* Match the term in Column I with the appropriate description in Column II.

COLUMN I		COLUMN II
A. Non-self substances	______.	Long-term immunity acquired following an infection or vaccination
B. Skin and mucous membranes	______.	Immediate hypersensitivity reaction that can be life-threatening
C. Active immunity	______.	Infectious microorganism
D. Passive immunity	______.	Immunity moderated by the link between T cells and phagocytic cells
E. Anaphylaxis	______.	Temporary immunity achieved by obtaining antibodies from another source (i.e., colostrum)
F. Cell-mediated immunity	______.	First infection barrier

CHAPTER 7 GENETICS, CONCEPTION, AND FETAL DEVELOPMENT

1. *Genetic Crossword*

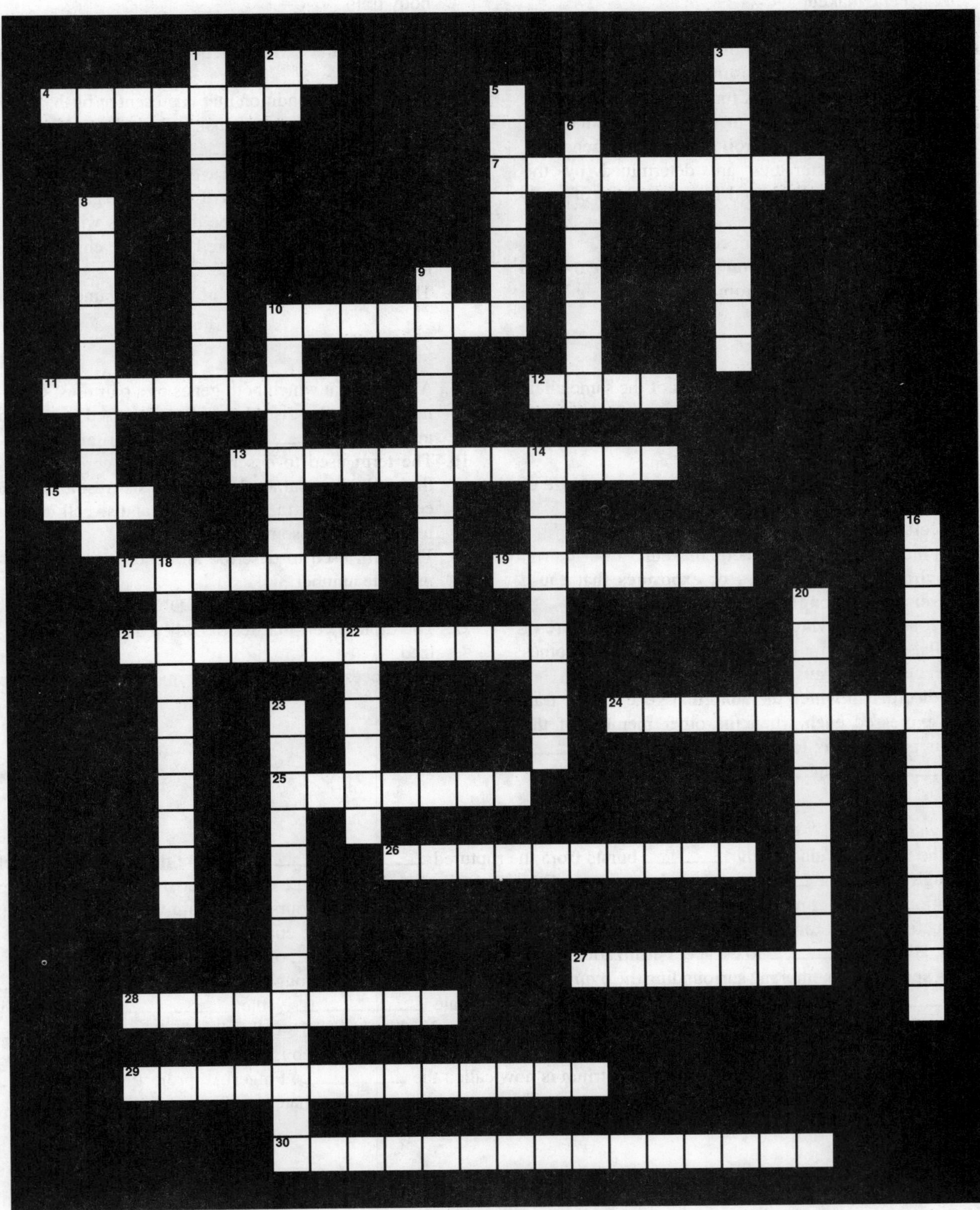

ACROSS:

2. The female sex chromosomes pair.
4. The product of the union of a normal gamete with a gamete containing an extra chromosome.
7. An individual's physical appearance as determined by genetic makeup.
10. A cell that contains 46 chromosomes.
11. The product of the union of a normal gamete with a gamete missing a chromosome.
12. A small segment of DNA found on chromosomes.
13. A pattern of inheritance in which a particular trait, disease, or defect is controlled by a single gene.
15. Physical characteristics are determined by this hereditary material carried in the nucleus of every cell.
17. The male and female germ cells.
19. The process of cell division used to produce ova and sperm that contain 23 chromosomes.
21. An individual who has two different alleles for a trait is said to be ____________ for that trait.
24. The 22 pairs of chromosomes that control most body traits.
25. The process by which a cell replicates, yielding two cells with the same genetic makeup as the parent cell.
26. An abnormal condition that is present at birth.
27. Inborn errors of metabolism reflect absent or defective ____________ to metabolize protein, fats, or carbohydrates.
28. The maturational process of the female gamete.
29. The term used to describe the process whereby genetic material is transferred from one chromosome to a different chromosome.
30. The maturational process of the male gamete.

DOWN:

1. An individual who has two copies of the same allele for a given trait is said to be ____________ for that trait.
2. The male sex chromosomes pair.
3. A pictorial analysis of the number, form, and size of an individual's chromosomes.
5. A cell that contains 23 single chromosomes.
6. An individual's entire genetic makeup.
8. Environmental substances or exposures that cause adverse effects on fetal development.
9. A condition in which an individual has a mixture of cells, some with a normal number of chromosomes and others with missing or extra chromosomes.
10. A disorder in which the abnormal gene for the trait is expressed even when the other member of the pair is normal is termed autosomal ____________ ____________ inheritance.
14. A disorder in which both genes of a pair must be abnormal for the disorder to be expressed is termed autosomal ____________ inheritance.
16. The term used to describe a pair of chromosomes that fails to separate during meiosis, resulting in a cell with an extra chromosome and a cell with a missing chromosome.
18. The term used to describe an abnormality of chromosome number.
20. Threadlike strands formed by DNA.
22. The diploid cell that results when an ovum is fertilized.
23. The process of maturation for male and female germ cells.

2. *Fill in the blanks.*

At the time of ovulation, the ________ bursts from the ruptured ________ . ________ capture the ovum and propel it through the uterine ________ toward the uterus. Ova are fertile for about ______ hours after ovulation. Following ejaculation, ________ reach the site of fertilization in an average of ________ hours and remain viable in a woman's reproductive system for ______ days. With the process of ________ the protective coating from the sperm heads is removed, allowing ________ to escape. Fertilization takes place in the ____________ of the uterine tube. Once penetrated by a sperm, the membrane surrounding the ovum becomes ____________ through a process termed the ________ — ____________ . With the fusion of the male and female ____________ , the ____________ number of chromosomes is restored. The new cell is called a ____________ . Within days, a 16-cell ball called the ____________ is formed. A cavity develops within this ball of cells, creating the ________ , which is ____________ into the endometrium days after conception. The endometrium is now called the ________ . Fingerlike projections called ____ ________ develop from the ____________ . These projections tap into maternal blood vessels in the decidua ________ .

3. The following structures play a critical role in fetal growth and development. List the functions of each.

   Yolk sac

   Amniotic membranes and fluid

   Umbilical cord

   Placenta

4. Fetal circulation differs from neonatal circulation. Describe the location and purpose of each of the following fetal circulatory structures:

   Ductus venosus liver

   Ductus arteriosus aorta/pulmonary

   Foramen ovale rt. atrium

5. Imagine that you are a nurse-midwife working in partnership with an obstetrician. How would you respond to each of the following concerns/questions directed to you from some of your prenatal clients?

   A. June (2 months pregnant), Mary (5 months pregnant), and Alice (7 months pregnant) each asks for a current description of her fetus.

      June Mary Alice

   B. Jessica states that a friend told her that babies born after about 35 weeks have a better chance to survive because they can breathe more easily. She asks if this is true.

   C. Beth, who is 1 month pregnant, states that she heard that women who are pregnant experience quickening. She wants to know what that could mean and if it hurts.

   D. Susan, who is 6 months pregnant, states that she read in a magazine that a fetus can actually hear and see. She feels that this is totally unbelievable.

   E. Alexa is 2 months pregnant. She asks how the sex of her baby was determined and if a sonogram could tell whether she was having a boy or a girl.

   F. Karen is pregnant for the first time. She reveals that she has a history of twins in her family. She wants to know what causes twin pregnancies to occur and what the difference is between identical and fraternal twins.

6. Mr. and Mrs. Goldberg are newly married and are planning for pregnancy. They express to the nurse their concern that Mrs. Goldberg has a history of Tay-Sachs disease in her family. Mr. Goldberg is unsure of his history. Briefly describe the process the nurse should follow in helping the Goldbergs determine their genetic risk and cope with an unsatisfactory outcome.

CHAPTER 8 ANATOMY AND PHYSIOLOGY OF PREGNANCY

1. Using the 5-digit system, describe the obstetric history for each of the following women:

   A. Jane is pregnant for the second time. Her first pregnancy resulted in a stillbirth at 36 weeks' gestation.

   B. May is 6 weeks pregnant. Her previous two pregnancies resulted in the live birth of a daughter at 40 weeks and a son at 41 weeks.

   C. Susan is experiencing her fourth pregnancy. Her first pregnancy ended in a spontaneous abortion at 8 weeks, the second resulted in the live birth of twin boys at 38 weeks, and the third resulted in the live birth of a daughter at 34 weeks.

2. *Matching:* Match the assessment data in Column I with the appropriate term in Column II.

COLUMN I	COLUMN II
A. Menstruation has ceased	______. Hegar's sign
B. Fundal height has decreased with fetal head engaged in pelvic inlet	______. Colostrum
C. Cervix and vagina are bluish	______. Braxton Hicks' sign
D. Softened, compressible uterine isthmus	______. Quickening
E. Softened cervix	______. Operculum
F. Irregular contractions of the uterus noted with abdominal palpation (painless)	______. Amenorrhea
G. Fetal head rebounds with gentle upward tapping through vagina	______. Pyrosis
H. Perception of "life" noted as a fluttering in the abdomen	______. Striae gravidarum
I. Thick, white vaginal discharge with a faint, musty odor	______. Linea nigra
J. Endocervical canal filled with plug of thick mucus	______. Ballottement
K. Reddish stretch marks noted on breasts and abdomen	______. Chadwick's sign
L. Thick, creamy fluid expressed from nipples	______. Lordosis
M. Cheeks, nose, and forehead blotchy and darker in appearance	______. Leukorrhea
N. Pigmented line on midline of abdomen	______. Chloasma
O. Small, red, raised nodules on gums	______. Lightening
P. Accentuated lumbosacral curve	______. Epulis
Q. "Acid indigestion" experienced after evening meal	______. Goodell's sign

3. How would you respond to each of the following client concerns/questions?

   A. Janet is 2 months pregnant. She calls the prenatal clinic to report that she noticed slight, painless spotting this morning. She states that she did have sex with her partner the night before.

   B. Alice suspects she is pregnant and is coming to the clinic tomorrow for a pregnancy test of her urine. She asks for instructions.

   C. Susan is 3 months pregnant. She tells you that she is worried because a friend told her that vaginal and bladder infections are more common during pregnancy. She wants to know if this could be true and, if so, why.

   D. Elise tells you that since she has been pregnant she has noted some "problems" with her breasts: there are "little pimples" near her nipples, and her breasts feel "lumpy and bumpy" when she does a BSE.

   E. Jean is concerned after reading in a book about pregnancy that a pregnant woman's position could affect her circulation, especially to the baby. She asks what are good positions for her now that she is pregnant.

   F. Angela, a pregnant woman, calls to tell you she had a nosebleed this morning and has noticed occasional feelings of fullness in her ears. She asks if these occurrences are anything to worry about.

   G. Karen is 7 months pregnant and works as a secretary full time. She asks you if she should take a "water pill" that a friend gave her, since she has noticed that her ankles "swell up" at the end of the day.

H. Marion is in her third trimester of pregnancy. She tells you that her posture seems to have changed and that she occasionally experiences low back pain.

I. Arlene is pregnant for the first time. She is worried, since her grandmother told her to expect to lose a tooth before the pregnancy is over. She tells you that she hopes it will not be one of her front teeth.

4. When assessing the pregnant woman, the nurse must be aware that baseline vital sign values will change as the woman progresses through her pregnancy (review this information in Chapter 8).

   A. Describe how each of the following would change:
      - Blood pressure
      - Heart rate and patterns
      - Respiratory rate and patterns
      - Body temperature

   B. Calculate the mean arterial pressure (MAP) for each of the following BP readings:
      - 120/76
      - 114/64
      - 130/80

5. Describe the value changes that occur in the following laboratory tests as a result of normal pregnancy adaptations.
   - CBC: Hematocrit (HCT) and hemoglobin (HG) White blood cell count (WBC)
   - Clotting activity
   - Acid/base balance
   - Urinalysis

6. Describe the expected changes in elimination that occur during pregnancy. Include in your answer the basis for the changes.

   Bladder

   Bowel

7. Explain why an increase in each of the following substances is critical for a healthy pregnancy outcome:

   A. Parathormone
   B. Insulinase
   C. Estrogen
   D. Progesterone
   E. Thyroxine
   F. Human chorionic gonadotropin (hCG)

CHAPTER 9 MATERNAL AND FETAL NUTRITION

1. Nutrition and weight gain are important areas of consideration for nurses who care for pregnant women. In addition, weight gain is often a source of stress and body image alteration for the pregnant woman. Discuss the approach you would use in each of the following situations.

   A. Alice (5 ft 8 in, 130 lb) complains to you that her physician recommended a weight gain of approximately 30 pounds during her pregnancy. She states, "Babies only weigh about 7 pounds when they are born! Why do I have to gain so much more than that?"

   B. Sharon (5 ft 4 in, 125 lb) has just found out that she is pregnant. She states, "I am so glad to be pregnant. I love to eat, and now I can start eating for two. It will be great not to have to watch the scale."

   C. Jane tells you that she does not have to worry about her nutrient intake during her pregnancy. "I take plenty of vitamins—everything from A to Z!"

   D. Mary is 6 months pregnant. She asks you if it is okay to take sodium bicarbonate for the heartburn she experiences after dinner.

   E. Alexa (BMI = 28.7) is 1 month pregnant. She asks you for dietary guidance, including a weight-reduction diet, since she does not want to gain too much more weight with this pregnancy.

2. Sara is an 18-year-old Native American woman (5 ft 6 in and 98 lb) who has just been diagnosed as 8 weeks pregnant. In her discussions with you at her first prenatal visit, she expresses an interest in learning about the nutritional requirements of pregnancy.

   A. Outline the approach that you would take in order to help her learn about and meet the nutritional needs of her pregnancy.

   B. Plan a two-day menu that incorporates Sara's individual nutritional needs.

3. For each of the following nutrients, state its importance for pregnancy and fetal development and the major food sources in which it can be found.

Nutrient	**Food sources**
Protein	
Fluids	
Iron	
Calcium	
Sodium	
Zinc	
Fat-soluble vitamins	
Water-soluble vitamins	

4. What concerns need to be addressed when caring for a client who is a vegan?

5. What guidance would you give to a client who has lactose intolerance?

6. Develop a plan of care that includes goals and interventions for each of the following nursing diagnoses:

   A. Alteration in nutrition: less than body requirements related to inadequate intake associated with moderate nausea and vomiting (morning sickness).

   Goals **Interventions**

   B. Knowledge deficit related to iron supplementation during pregnancy.

   Goals **Interventions**

CHAPTER 10 FAMILY DYNAMICS OF PREGNANCY

1. Using the framework of crisis and crisis intervention, as presented in Chapter 2 (pp. 30 to 32), discuss:

   A. How pregnancy meets the criteria of a maturational crisis.

   B. The crisis intervention measures you would use to help the pregnant woman and her family to meet the demands of this maturational change with a minimal degree of stress and anxiety.

2. Your neighbor, Jane Smith, is in her second month of pregnancy. Knowing that you are a nurse, her husband Tom confides in you that he just cannot "figure Jane out. One minute she is happy and the next minute she is crying for no reason at all! I do not know how I will be able to cope with this for 7 more months." How would you respond to his concern?

3. Your friend Mary is 7 months pregnant. She tells you that she is very concerned about her husband's behavior. She states, "He has been working overtime every week and is even considering a part-time job on the weekends. He told me he does not know how he will be able to fit the Lamaze classes in his schedule or if he even will be good at it." What would you tell her?

4. Body image changes and concerns may be profound for a pregnant woman. Briefly discuss each of the following:

   A. The changes that occur and how they can affect a pregnant woman and her partner.

   B. The nursing measures that could be used to assist an expectant couple as they attempt to deal with body changes during pregnancy in a positive manner.

5. Susan, a primigravida at 8 weeks' gestation, confides in you that most of the time she is happy to be pregnant, but sometimes "I am so mad at my baby for making me feel sick to my stomach and too tired to concentrate on my job. Is this a sign that I will be a bad mother?" How would you respond to her concern?

6. Grandparents should be considered when working with expectant families.

   A. Describe the role that grandparents play in the pregnancies of their children and the success of their transition to parenthood.

   B. How could you, as a nurse, assist grandparents in their adaptation to their children's pregnancy?

7. Jim's partner Mary is 5 months pregnant. He tells you that sometimes he feels "left out" of Mary's pregnancy and asks you if he is important to Mary as her partner and the father of the baby. How would you answer his question?

8. A nurse-midwife tells Mrs. Orlando that she is pregnant. After discussing some of the changes to expect during pregnancy, Mrs. Orlando shyly asks how pregnancy could affect her "sex life" with her husband. "It has been so good; what if it changes?" How should the nurse-midwife respond?

9. Describe the three developmental tasks/phases that must be completed by an expectant couple during their transition to parenthood.

	Mother	**Father**
Phase I		
Phase II		
Phase III		

10. Pregnant couples often prepare a birth plan during the third trimester of pregnancy.

    A. What is a birth plan, and what purpose does it serve?

    B. What can a nurse learn from a couple's birth plan?

    C. How should the nurse use the birth plan when providing care for the laboring couple?

11. Jane is 4 months pregnant and beginning to "show." She asks you what she should expect as a reaction from her 4-year-old daughter and techniques that she could use to help her child adapt in a positive manner. Describe your response.

CHAPTER 11 FIRST TRIMESTER

1. *Matching:* Match the assessment data in Column I with the appropriate designation from Column II.

COLUMN I	COLUMN II
____. Striae gravidarum	A. Presumptive symptom
____. Breast tenderness	B. Presumptive sign
____. Enlarged abdomen	C. Probable sign
____. Amenorrhea	D. Positive sign
____. Fetal movement noted by examiner	
____. Fatigue	
____. Chloasma	
____. Quickening	
____. Elevated fundus	
____. Periodic nausea with vomiting	
____. Uterine souffle	
____. Braxton Hicks' sign	
____. Chadwick's sign	
____. Fetal heart tones	
____. Positive home pregnancy test	
____. Goodell's sign	

2. Using Nägele's rule, calculate the expected date of delivery (EDD) for each of the following pregnant women:

   A. Mary's last menses began on May 20, 1993, and its last day occurred on May 25, 1993.

   B. Susan had intercourse on February 12, 1993. She has not had a menstrual period since the one that began on January 24, 1993, and ended 5 days later.

   C. Dawn has regular 32-day cycles. Her last period began on September 4, 1993, and ended on September 8, 1993.

3. Imagine that you are a nurse working in a prenatal clinic. You have been assigned to be the primary nurse for Susan, an 18-year-old who has come to the clinic for confirmation of pregnancy. She tells you that she knows she is pregnant because she has already missed 3 periods and a home pregnancy test that she did last week was positive. Susan states that she has had very little contact with health care, and the only reason she came today is because her boyfriend insisted that she "make sure" she is really pregnant. Describe the approach that you would take regarding data collection and nursing intervention appropriate for this client.

4. During a prenatal examination of a pregnant client, it is important to determine her level of knowledge and ability with regard to BSE. Describe how you would evaluate the client in this regard and the criteria you would use as part of this evaluation.

5. Janet has come to your clinic for diagnosis of a possible pregnancy. As part of the assessment, a pelvic examination will be performed by the physician. Janet tells you that she has never had this type of examination before. As the nurse who will be with her, how would you help Janet cope with this examination and make it a positive experience?

6. During a prenatal pelvic and genital examination, specimens are obtained for a variety of laboratory tests. Identify these tests, and describe their purpose and importance during pregnancy.

7. For each of the following situations, write a nursing diagnosis. Based on the nursing diagnosis you have identified, list goals and interventions that would be appropriate.

   A. Mary is 6 weeks pregnant. During the health history interview, she tells you that she has limited her intake of fluids and tries to hold her urine as long as she can because "I just do not have the time to keep going to the bathroom."

NURSING DIAGNOSIS	GOALS	INTERVENTIONS

   B. Angela is in her first trimester of pregnancy. She works long hours as a secretary and plans to continue to the last week or two of her pregnancy. When she gets home, she is usually so tired that she sits around and watches TV after supper. Now that she is pregnant she wants to become more active, since she heard it is good for her and the baby. But, as she tells you, "I just do not know how to get started or what kinds of activity would be okay."

NURSING DIAGNOSIS	GOALS	INTERVENTIONS

8. Cultural beliefs and practices are important influencing factors during the prenatal period.

   A. Describe how cultural beliefs can affect a woman's participation in prenatal care as it is defined by the western biomedical model of care.

   B. Identify one **prescription** and one **proscription** for each of the following areas:

      - Emotional responses
      - Clothing
      - Physical activity and rest
      - Sexual activity
      - Dietary practices (refer to Chapter 9)

CHAPTER 12 SECOND TRIMESTER

1. Briefly discuss why emotional well-being must be assessed and considered at every prenatal visit.

2. Which of the following second-trimester pregnant women exhibits a risk for pregnancy-induced hypertension (PIH)? Review Chapter 8 as necessary.

CLIENT	BASELINE BLOOD PRESSURE	CURRENT BLOOD PRESSURE
Mary	120/70	130/80
Janice	100/60	130/68
Susan	115/70	120/66
Marie	122/86	126/70

A. Identify the criteria that you used to determine risk.

B. Identify three factors that can influence the accuracy of a BP measurement.

3. Answer each of the following questions asked by Alice, a primigravida, during a second-trimester prenatal visit.

A. "Why do you measure my abdomen every time I come in for a checkup?"
B. How can you tell if my baby is doing okay?"
C. "I have always enjoyed a glass or two of wine with dinner. I stopped during my first 3 months because I know babies can be affected early in pregnancy. Now that I am 14 weeks along, is it okay to have just one glass a day?"
D. "I am going to start changing the way that I dress now that I am beginning to show. Do you have any suggestions I could follow, especially since I have a limited amount of money to spend?"
E. "What can I do about gas? I never had much of a problem before I was pregnant."
F. "I wear a seat belt now, but should I still do so when my abdomen gets a little bigger?"

4. Using McDonald's rule, estimate the gestational age in weeks and lunar months for each of the following fundal heights:

16 cm 20 cm 24 cm

Identify the steps a nurse can take to ensure more accurate fundal measurements.

5. For each of the following situations, write one nursing diagnosis. Based on the nursing diagnosis you have identified, list goals and interventions that would be appropriate.

A. Mary, who is 23 weeks pregnant, tells you that she is beginning to experience more frequent lower back pain. You note that when she walked into the examining room her posture exhibited a moderate degree of lordosis, and she was wearing shoes with 2-inch narrow heels.

NURSING DIAGNOSES	GOALS	INTERVENTIONS

B. Susan is 20 weeks pregnant. Her obstetric history using the 5-digit system is 3-0-1-1-0. You observe that her anxiety level has been increasing gradually. She states that she is afraid of losing another baby and just does not know what she can do to keep herself and her baby healthy.

NURSING DIAGNOSES	GOALS	INTERVENTIONS

CHAPTER 13 THIRD TRIMESTER

1. Allison is a primigravida at 36 weeks' gestation. Indicate which of the following signs/symptoms, if present, would indicate a potential complication of pregnancy. For each of the signs/symptoms listed, state its physiologic basis.

SIGNS/SYMPTOMS	PHYSIOLOGIC BASIS
____ A. Urinary frequency	
____ B. Blurred vision	
____ C. Inability to remove rings	
____ D. Abdominal cramps with diarrhea	
____ E. Infrequent, irregular uterine contractions	
____ F. Occasional, mild headaches	
____ G. Insomnia	
____ H. Dysuria	
____ I. Nonpitting ankle edema	
____ J. Small amount of clear, watery discharge from vagina	
____ K. Feelings of jitteriness	

2. *True or False:* Circle "T" if true or "F" if false for each of the following statements. Correct the false statements.

T F During the third trimester, a pregnant woman's attention toward securing safe passage may include fears of pain, mutilation, and loss of control during labor.

T F A roll-over test is said to be positive if the systolic blood pressure decreases by 15 mm Hg when the pregnant woman changes from a lateral to a supine position.

T F It is necessary that every expectant couple develop a birth plan and attend childbirth education classes.

T F A new immunization strategy being investigated is to protect newborns from *Haemophilus influenzae* type B by vaccinating their mothers during the third trimester.

T F RhoGAM is administered at about 28 weeks' gestation to pregnant women who are Rh_o, D negative with a positive Coombs' test result.

T F A definitive sign of preterm labor would be uterine contractions occurring every 15 minutes or four times in 1 hour.

T F The primary goal of childbirth preparation classes is a pain-free labor and birth.

T F Each expectant father needs to actively participate in the birth of his child by coaching his partner during labor and birth.

T F Monozygotic twins are more likely to develop congenital anomalies and two-vessel umbilical cords than dizygotic twins or singletons.

3. Following a sonogram, Anna (2-1-0-0-1) and her husband were told that they are going to have twins. They ask you how this pregnancy may differ from their first pregnancy, which was a singleton pregnancy.

4. Jennifer (2-1-0-0-1) and her husband Dan are beginning their third trimester of an uncomplicated pregnancy. As you work with them on their birth plan, they tell you that they have narrowed down their choice of a birth setting to a local free-standing birth center or their own home, since their first pregnancy was "perfectly normal from start to finish." They seek information from you so that they can make the right decision. Describe how you would counsel them in their decision-making process.

5. Women often fear the pain that will accompany childbirth.

   A. Describe the potentially harmful effects of the pain experienced in childbirth.

   B. Briefly describe how each of the following nonpharmacologic methods could be useful for pain relief during labor and birth:

      Gate control techniques

      Relaxation methods

      Paced breathing techniques

      Biofeedback

      Therapeutic touch

      Acupressure

      Imagery

      Music

CHAPTER 14 ESSENTIAL FACTORS AND PROCESSES OF LABOR

1. Label the following illustrations of the fetal skull and the maternal pelvis with the appropriate landmarks and diameters. Include the average measurement of each of the fetal skull and maternal pelvic diameters.

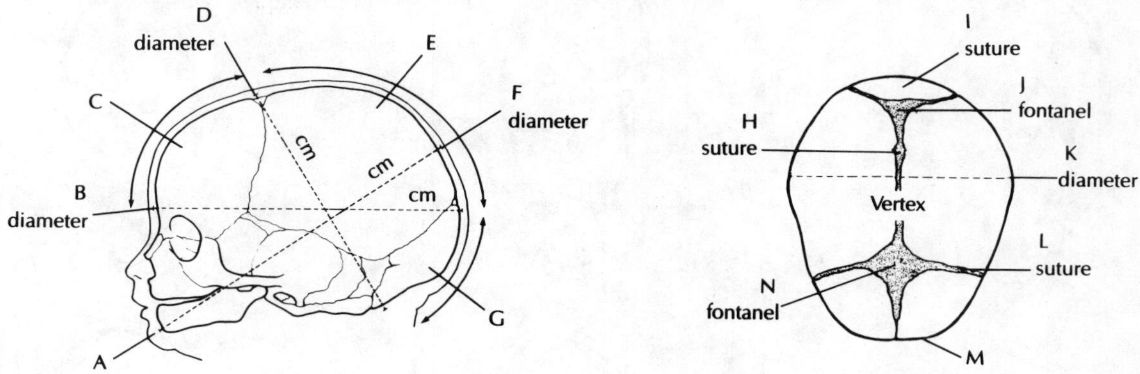

FETAL SKULL

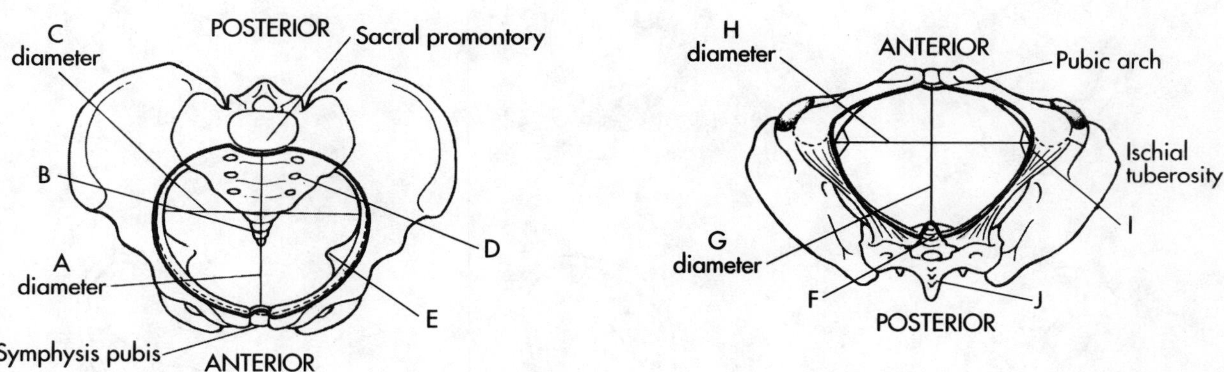

MATERNAL PELVIS

2. For each of the following illustrations, indicate the presentation, presenting part, position, lie, and attitude of the fetus.

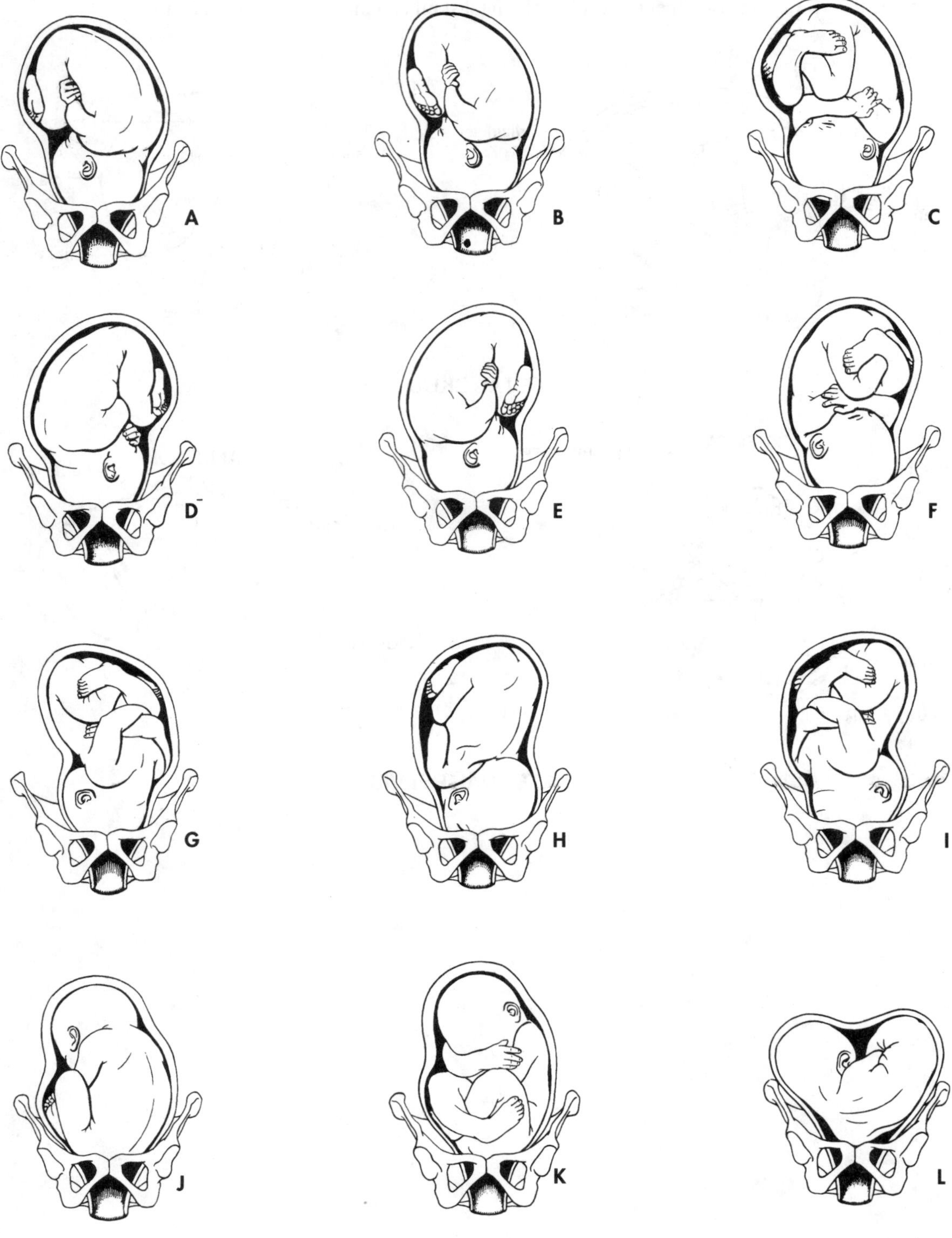

3. Identify and briefly describe the five P's of labor. Include in your description the manner in which each factor facilitates the progress of labor and birth.

4. As part of their care of the laboring woman, nurses perform vaginal examinations and interpret the results. State the meaning of each of the following vaginal examination findings:

EXAM I	EXAM II	EXAM III	EXAM IV
ROP	RMA	LST	QO
−1		+1	+3
50%	25%	75%	100%
3 cm	2 cm	6 cm	10 cm

5. Mary is a primigravida at 36 weeks' gestation. During her prenatal visit, she asks you the following questions regarding her approaching labor. How would you respond?

   A. "What gets labor started?"

   B. "Are there things I should watch for that would indicate that my labor is getting closer to starting?"

6. ***A Labor and Birth Crossword***

ACROSS:

2. The stage of labor during which the cervix widens and thins.
4. The cardinal movement of labor to facilitate the emergence of the fetal head.
5. The third stage of labor is also known as the ______ ______ stage.
7. The level of the __________ ____________ is station zero.
9. Overlapping of the fetal skull bones to facilitate its passage through the bony pelvis.
12. "Dropping" of the fetal presenting part into the true pelvis.
14. The presenting part of a cephalic presentation when the head is fully flexed.
16. Term that refers to the part of the fetus that enters the pelvic inlet first.
18. The smallest anteroposterior diameter of the fetal skull.
20. Relationship of the fetal body parts to each other.
21. Softening of the cervix in preparation for labor's onset.
22. The ____________ fontanelle lies at the junction of the sagittal and lambdoid sutures.
24. Another term used for the anterior fontanelle.
25. When the cervix shortens and thins, it is said to __________.
27. The series of events that occur before the onset of true labor is termed _________ labor.
30. Contraction of abdominal muscles and diaphragm as the secondary powers of labor.
31. For birth to occur, the fetus must accommodate to this rigid passageway.
33. Relationship of the fetal spine to the maternal spine.
34. Rotation maneuver to allow the fetal head to pass through the pelvic outlet is termed ___________ rotation.
35. The time between the beginning of one uterine contraction and the beginning of the next.
36. When the cervical os widens or opens it is said to ____.
37. Strength of a uterine contraction.
38. Length of a uterine contraction.

DOWN:

1. The cardinal movement of labor that occurs as the fetal shoulders engage and descend through the pelvis is termed ___________ rotation.
3. The stage of labor when the fetus is born.
6. Passage of cervical mucous plug before the onset of labor is termed ____________ show.
8. Measurement of fetal descent in relationship to the ischial spines.
9. Presenting part of a cephalic presentation when the fetal head is in extension.
10. The stage of recovery following birth of the placenta.
11. Head-first presentation.
13. The most common form of pelvis for the female.
15. A labor curve.
17. Realignment of the fetal head with its back and shoulders after the head is born.
19. Presenting part in a buttocks-first presentation.
22. Uterine contractions.
23. Buttocks-first presentation.
26. Cardinal movement of labor that permits the smallest anteroposterior diameter of the fetal skull to pass through the pelvis.
27. Relationship of the presenting part to the four quadrants of the maternal pelvis.
28. Suture located between the two parietal bones of the fetal skull.
29. Downward progress of the presenting part through the pelvis.
32. When the biparietal diameter of the fetal head passes through the pelvic inlet, it is said to be ___________.

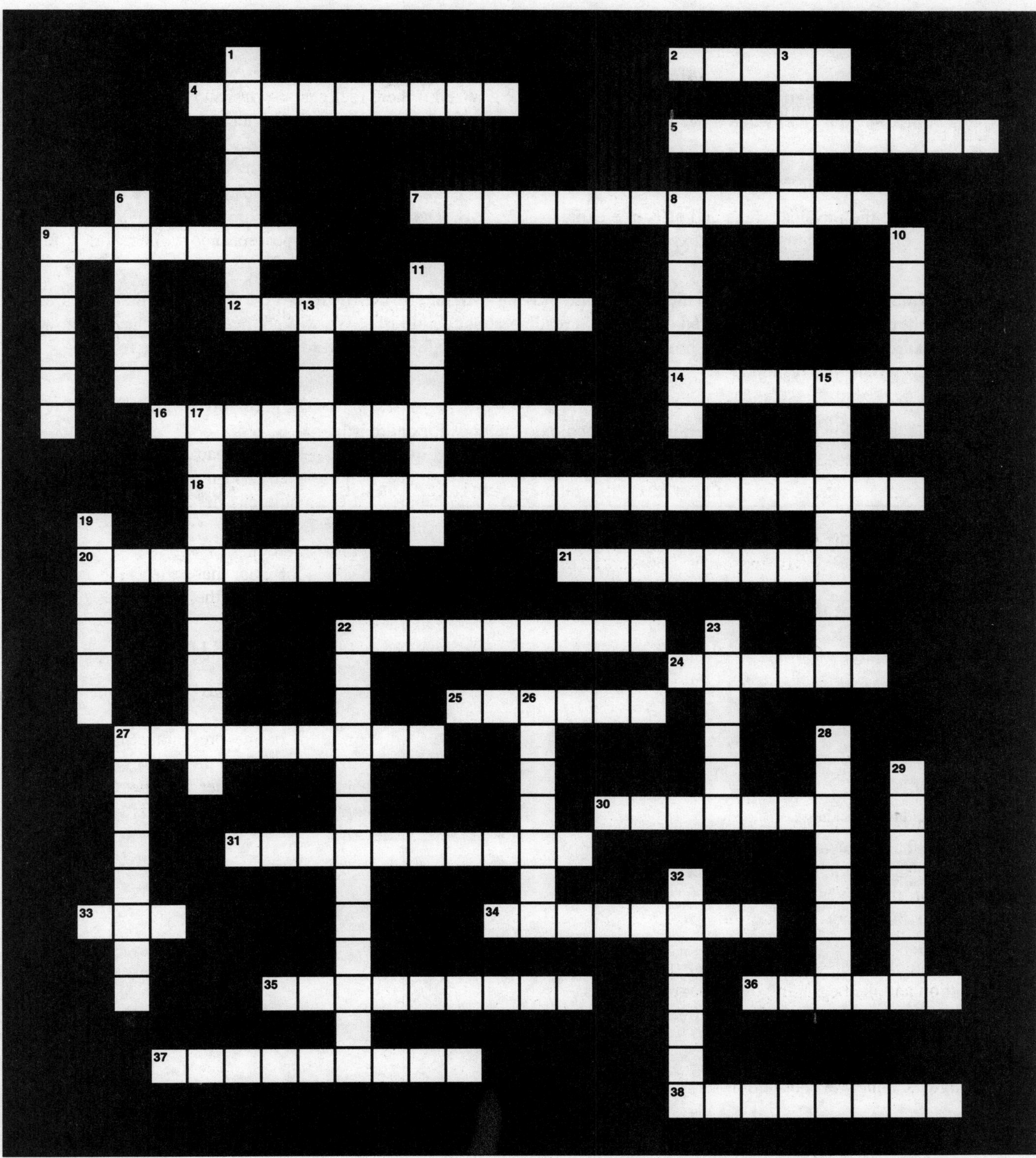

CHAPTER 15 PHARMACOLOGIC MANAGEMENT OF DISCOMFORT

1. When working with a group of expectant fathers, the nurse is asked if there really is "a physical reason for all the pain women say they feel when they are in labor." Describe the response that this nurse should give.

2. Nurses working on labor and birth units must be sensitive to their clients' pain experiences.

   A. What are the physical signs and affective expressions of pain that nurses would expect to see?

   B. Describe specific measures nurses could use to alter their clients' perception of pain.

3. Upon admission to the labor unit in the latent phase of labor, Mr. and Mrs. Brown (2-0-0-1-0) tell you that they are so glad they took Lamaze classes and did so much reading about childbirth. "We will not need any medication now that we know what to do. But most importantly, our baby will be safe!" If you were their primary nurse for childbirth, how would you respond?

4. Complete the following table concerning pharmacologic methods for childbirth:

METHOD	EFFECTS	CRITERIA FOR USE	NURSING MANAGEMENT
Sedatives			
Systemic Analgesics			
Narcotics			
Mixed narcotics			
Narcotic antagonists			
Ataractics			
Nerve Blocks			
Pudendal			
Spinal anesthetic			
Lumbar epidural anesthesia			
Lumbar epidural analgesia			
General Anesthesia			

CHAPTER 16 FETAL MONITORING

1. It is critical that a nurse working on a labor unit be knowledgeable concerning factors associated with a reduction in fetal oxygen supply, characteristics of a reassuring FHR pattern, and characteristics of normal uterine activity. List the required information for each of the following:

   A. Factors associated with a reduction in fetal O_2 supply

   B. Characteristics of a reassuring FHR pattern

   C. Characteristics of normal uterine activity

2. Susan, a primigravida in active labor, has just been admitted to the labor unit. She becomes very anxious when the electronic monitoring equipment is set up. She tells the nurse that her father had a heart attack 2 months ago. "He was so sick they had to put him on a monitor, too. Does this mean that my baby has a heart problem like his grandfather?" How should the nurse respond?

3. Janet is a primigravida at 42 weeks' gestation. Her labor is being stimulated with oxytocin administered intravenously. Her moderate contractions are occurring every 3 minutes and last 60 seconds. She is currently in a supine position with a 30° elevation of her head. On observation of the monitor tracing, you note that during the last contraction the FHR decreased after the contraction peaked and did not return to baseline until about 15 seconds into the rest period. Variability and baseline rate appeared to be unaffected.

   A. Identify the pattern described and the possible factors responsible for it.

   B. Describe the actions you would take in order of priority. State the rationale for each action.

4. Discuss the nursing measures that can be used with the client who is in labor to prevent the occurrence of nonreassuring and ominous FHR patterns.

5. *Matching:* Match the FHR assessment data in Column I with the appropriate term in Column II (NOTE: each term may be used only once).

COLUMN I	COLUMN II
____. Average rate of 130 to 136 as determined between uterine contractions	A. Early deceleration
____. Persistent rate of 84 to 90 with minimal variability and frequent late decelerations	B. Variability
____. Persistent rate of 164 to 170	C. Late deceleration
____. Acceleration of FHR noted with fetal movement	D. Variable deceleration
____. Over the course of 1 minute the FHR ranged from 128 to 136 with four rhythmic cycles from baseline	E. Ominous pattern
____. FHR decreased shortly after onset of contraction with recovery as contraction ended	F. Nonreassuring pattern
____. FHR decreased after peak of contraction with recovery 20 seconds into rest period	G. Reassuring pattern
____. U-shaped FHR deceleration pattern noted following rupture of the membranes	H. Baseline FHR

6. State the advantages and disadvantages/limitations of each of the following monitoring techniques:

TECHNIQUE	ADVANTAGES	DISADVANTAGES/LIMITATIONS
Periodic auscultation		
EXTERNAL MONITORING: Ultrasound transducer		
Tocotransducer		
INTERNAL MONITORING: Spiral electrode		
Intrauterine catheter		

7. Evaluate each of the following monitor tracings using the FHR assessment checklist found in this chapter. Based on your assessment, describe the FHR pattern observed as reassuring, nonreassuring, or ominous. Include the nursing actions you would take based on your findings.

A.

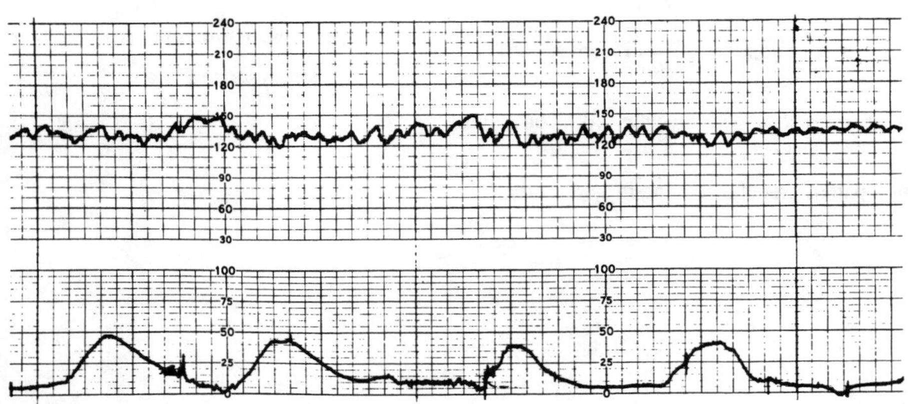

B.

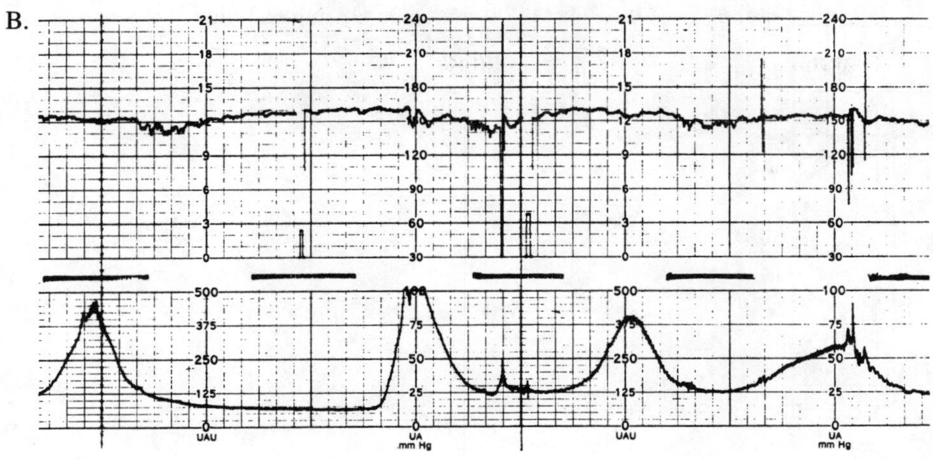

C.

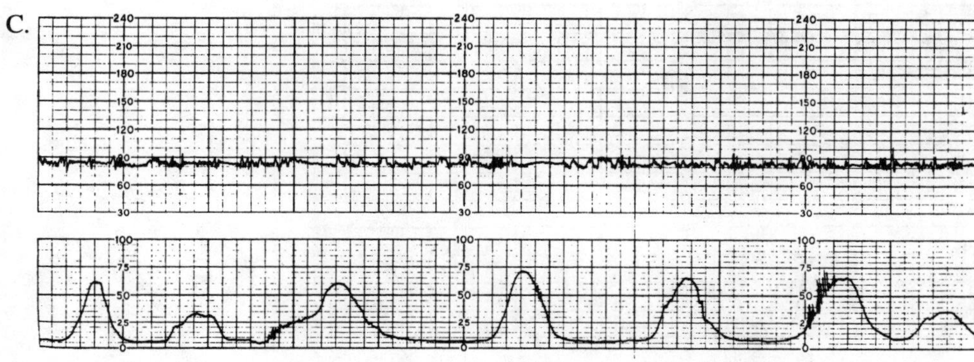

D.

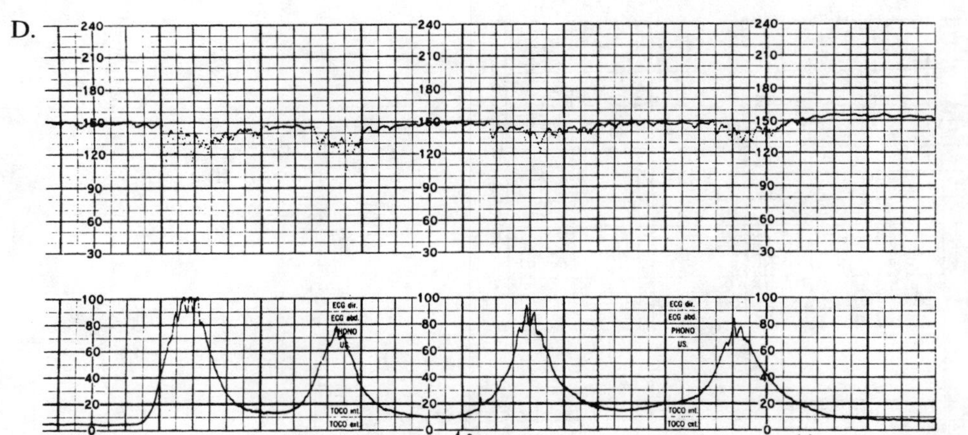

E.

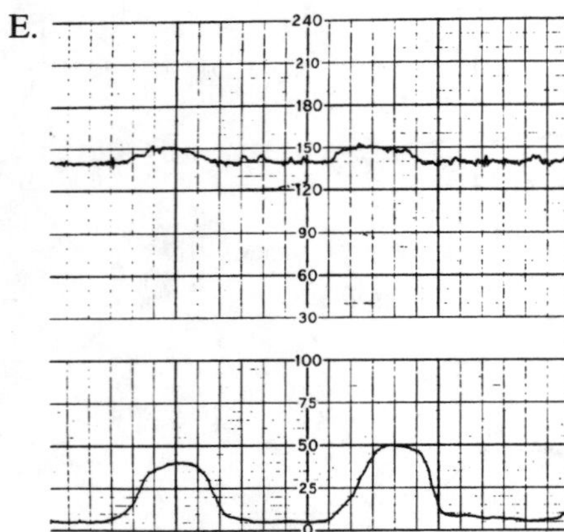

F.

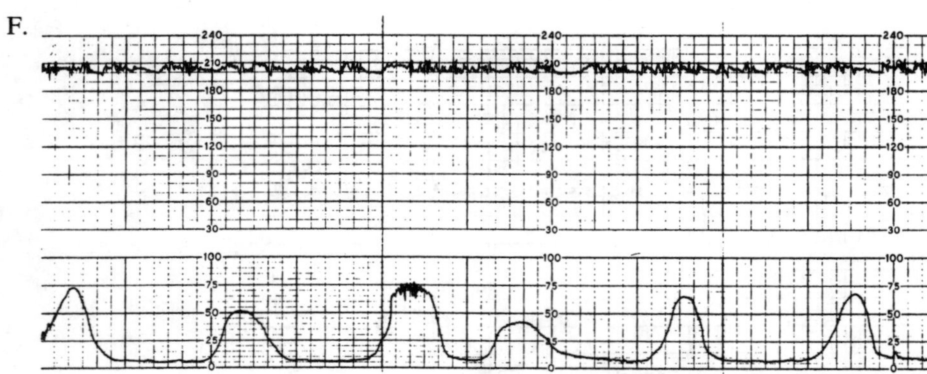

G.

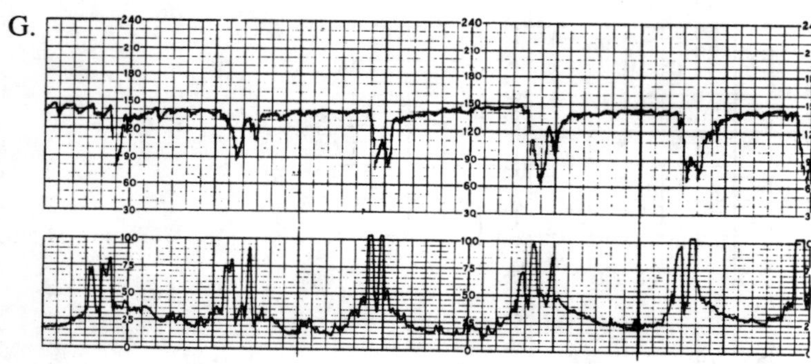

H.

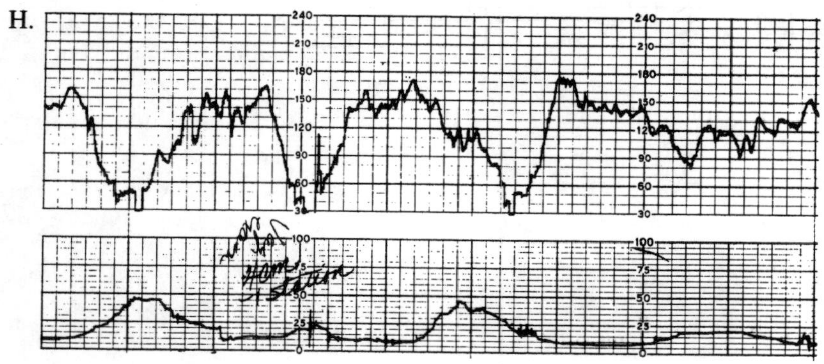

CHAPTER 17 FIRST STAGE OF LABOR

1. Evaluate each of the following signs and symptoms used in distinguishing true labor from false labor. Designate whether the sign/symptom is typical of *true labor* (1) or *false labor* (2).

   A. Contractions regular and progressive ____
   B. Cervix soft and posterior ____
   C. Contractions cease with ambulation ____
   D. Cervix, soft, 25%, 2 cm, midposition ____
   E. Lightening present in multiparous woman ____
   F. Discomfort present in abdomen above umbilicus ____
   G. Contraction intensity increases with activity and ambulation ____
   H. Presenting part at −2 station ____
   I. Bloody show ____
   J. Discomfort radiates from lower back to lower quadrants of abdomen ____

2. Martha calls the labor unit. She tells the nurse that she thinks she is in labor. "I have had some pains for about 2 hours." Describe how the nurse should approach this situation.

3. Susan (3-1-1-0-1) has just been admitted in latent labor. As part of the admission procedure you review her prenatal record, which also includes her obstetric history. List the data you would need to obtain from this record to plan care that is appropriate for Susan.

4. Describe the psychosocial support measures that would be appropriate for each of the following women in the first stage of their labor.

SUSAN	ALICE	DEBRA
6 cm	8 cm	2 cm
moderate	strong	mild
q4min	q3min	q6-7min
35-40 sec	50-60 sec	25-30 sec
0	+2	−1

5. Describe the method that should be used for applying an external FHR monitor (sonometer) to the abdomen of a laboring woman. Include the rationale for using this method.

6. Nancy, a woman in active labor, begins to cry during a vaginal examination to assess her status. "Why not watch the monitor to see how I am doing instead of doing these vaginal exams? They really hurt!"

   A. How should the nurse respond to Nancy's concern?

   B. Describe the measures the nurse should use to meet Nancy's safety and comfort needs during a vaginal examination.

7. Label the following illustration that depicts the characteristics of uterine contractions.

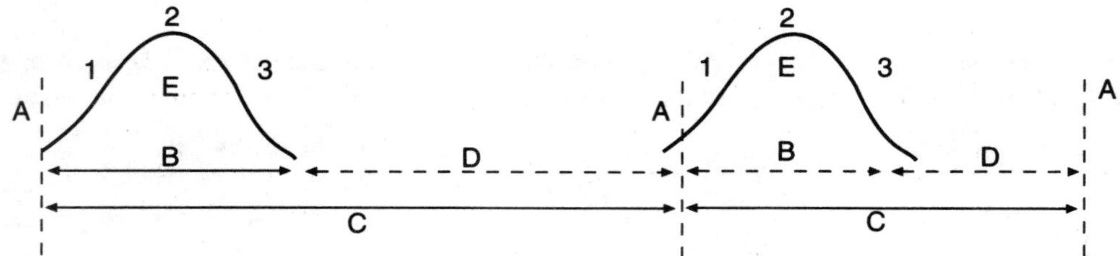

Describe how you would assess each of these characteristics using the palpation method.

8. Ann is 7 cm dilated. Her husband comes to tell you that her "water just broke with a gush!"

   A. In order of priority, describe each action you would take in this situation. Include the rationale for the actions you have identified.

   B. On evaluation a prolapse is noted, with the umbilical cord protruding slightly from the vagina. Describe your immediate actions, including rationale.

9. Mary, a 17-year-old primigravida, is admitted in the latent phase of labor. Her boyfriend Tom is with her as her only support. They appear committed to each other. During the admission interview, Mary tells you that they did not go to any classes because she was embarrassed about not being married. Both Mary and Tom appear very nervous, and assessment indicates they know little about what is happening, what to expect, and how to work together with the process of labor. Identify the nursing diagnoses reflected in this data. List the goals and nursing interventions appropriate for the diagnoses identified.

NURSING DIAGNOSES	GOALS	INTERVENTIONS

CHAPTER 18 SECOND AND THIRD STAGES OF LABOR

1. Marie (4-3-0-0-3) is in latent labor and is being oriented to the birthing room. Both she and her husband are amazed by the room and the birthing bed that will allow her to give birth in an upright position. They also are informed that changes in bearing-down efforts now allow a woman to follow her own body feelings and even to vocalize with pushing. Both Marie and her husband state that with every other birth they put her legs in stirrups, she held her breath for as long as she could, and pushed quietly. "Everything turned out okay—why should we change?" If you were the primary nurse for this couple, how would you respond to their concern?

2. *True or false:* Circle "T" if true or "F" if false for each of the following statements. Correct the false statements.

T F For childbirth to progress safely, a woman's bearing-down efforts must be carefully regulated.

T F The only certain objective sign of the onset of the second stage of labor is full dilatation and effacement of the cervix.

T F Absence of FHR variability is to be expected during the mother's bearing-down efforts.

T F During the second stage of labor, contractions and FHR are assessed every 10 minutes by evaluating the monitor tracing.

T F During the descent phase, pressure of the presenting part on the pelvic floor stimulates release of oxytocin from the pituitary gland, thus intensifying uterine contractions.

T F During birth of the head the woman must control her urge to push by taking panting breaths.

T F The duration of the second stage of labor for a nulliparous woman should not exceed 2 hours.

T F If stirrups are used during birth, it is important to place the left leg in its stirrup first.

T F The time of birth is recorded as the time when the entire fetal body has emerged from the mother.

T F After an emergency home birth of a live newborn, the umbilical cord should be cut as soon as possible to prevent newborn hemorrhage.

T F The priority goal for a newborn in the immediate postnatal period is that the newborn's airway remains patent.

T F The Apgar score is performed once after birth.

T F An erythromycin ointment is instilled into a newborn's eyes within 2 hours of birth to prevent eye inflammation caused by gonorrheal or chlamydial infection.

T F A side-lying position for childbirth is associated with a lower incidence of episiotomies.

3. Identify two support measures you would use during each of the phases of the second stage of labor. Validate your response with events and behavior typical of that phase.

PHASE	EVENTS/BEHAVIOR	SUPPORT MEASURES
Latent/resting		
Descent		
Final/transition		

4. A nurse living in a rural area is called to her neighbor's home to assist his wife who is in labor. "Everything is happening so fast—she says she is ready to deliver!" After the birth of a live newborn boy, what should the nurse do to prevent maternal hemorrhage until the ambulance arrives?

5. Placental separation and expulsion are the major events of the third stage of labor.

   A. Describe the process of placental separation.
   B. List the signs that indicate separation has occurred.
   C. Describe what the nurse should do to assist a woman to expel the placenta.

6. Angela has just given birth to a baby boy.

   A. Identify five priority assessments that must be made at this time to determine the newborn's status in terms of physiologic integrity.
   B. Identify measures used to promote neonatal physiologic integrity. State the rationale for the measures identified.
   C. Identify three measures that can be used to encourage parent-newborn attachment.

CHAPTER 19 FOURTH STAGE OF LABOR

1. Marion is 30 minutes into her fourth stage of labor after the birth of a full-term, living female. She complains that it hurts when the nurse pushes into her abdomen and asks her not to do it anymore.

   A. How should the nurse respond to Marion's concern?

   B. Describe the technique that the nurse should use to assess the fundus and to ensure the accuracy of the findings obtained.

   C. What characteristics regarding the fundus should be documented?

   D. When and how should the nurse perform fundal massage?

2. Describe the influence of a full bladder on the uterus during the stage of recovery.

3. Angela has a midline episiotomy, which the nurse must assess.

   A. What position should Angela assume to facilitate the examination of her episiotomy?

   B. Describe how the REEDA system can be used to assess and describe the episiotomy.

4. Anne gave birth 2 hours ago. On palpation her fundus was found to be 2 fingers above the umbilicus and deviated to the right. It also was found to be less firm than previously noted.

   A. What is the most likely cause for these findings?

   B. On the basis of these findings, what actions should be taken by the nurse?

5. The physician has written the following order: OOB (out of bed) 2 hours after birth. Describe the process you would use to safely fulfill this order.

6. Mary gave birth 1½ hours ago. She tells you that she is ravenous. You check the chart, noting the physician's order for "diet as tolerated." What criteria should be met before fulfilling this order?

7. Susan is a primigravida in the fourth stage of labor. She seems disinterested in her baby and asks if you would take him back to the nursery.

   A. What factors could account for her actions?

   B. What nursing measures could you use to encourage future maternal-newborn interaction?

8. Contrast normal fourth-stage signs and symptoms with those that could indicate hemorrhage and hypovolemic shock.

Expected signs/symptoms	Signs/symptoms that suggest hypovolemic shock

9. *Matching:* Match the description in Column I with the appropriate term in Column II.

COLUMN I	COLUMN II	
A. Uterine discharge typical of the fourth stage of labor	______.	Involution
B. Discomfort related to postpartum uterine contractions	______.	Atony
C. Reversal of the anatomic and physiologic adaptations to pregnancy	______.	Bradycardia
D. Blood clot formation at the site of the episiotomy	______.	Ecchymosis
E. Slowing of the pulse rate in response to cardiovascular changes after birth	______.	Orthostatic hypotension
F. Relaxation of the fundus	______.	Lochia rubra
G. Bruise on the perineum	______.	Afterpains
H. Causative factor for feeling lightheaded/dizzy when getting OOB for the first time after the birth	______.	Hematoma

CHAPTER 20 ASSESSMENT OF THE NEWBORN

1. Neonatal nurses are responsible for the assessment of a newborn's physiologic integrity. As part of this responsibility the nurse must be aware of the significance of data that are collected. Label each of the following assessment findings, if present in a 12-hour-old full-term male neonate, as "N" (reflective of normal adaptation to extrauterine life) or "P" (reflective of potential problems with adaptation to extrauterine life).

ASSESSMENT FINDING	EVALUATION
A. Crackles on auscultation of the lungs	___
B. Respirations: 36, irregular, shallow	___
C. Episodic apnea lasting 5 to 10 seconds	___
D. Slight bluish discoloration of feet	___
E. Jaundice on face and chest	___
F. Regurgitation after 8 AM feeding	___
G. Nasal flaring and slight sternal retraction	___
H. Head 34 cm and chest 36 cm	___
I. Apical rate: 126 with sinus arrhythmia	___
J. Overlapping of parietal bones	___
K. Hematocrit 36% and hemoglobin 12 g	___
L. Liver palpated 1 cm below right costal margin	___
M. Spine straight with dimple at base	___
N. Slightly depressed anterior fontanelle	___
O. Adhesion of prepuce—unable to fully retract	___

2. Respiration, circulation, and heat regulation are the three factors most crucial to the newborn's extrauterine existence. Describe the interrelationship of these survival factors.

RESPIRATION	CIRCULATION	THERMOGENESIS

3. *Fill in the blanks:*

Variations in state of consciousness of newborn infants are called the __________ - __________ cycles. There are ____ sleep states and ____ wake states. The optimum state of arousal is the ____ ____ state, in which the infant can be observed smiling, vocalizing, and moving in synchrony. In the ______ ______ state the infant is more sensitive to hunger, fatigue, and noise. The newborn sleeps about ______ hours a day. In ______ sleep the newborn is nearly still except for occasional spontaneous startles or twitches. On the other hand, ______ sleep is characterized by the presence of REMS.

4. Significant differences occur in the physiologic functioning of the newborn and the adult. Fill in the following table, which relates to these differences and the implications for newborn care.

PHYSIOLOGIC FUNCTION	NEWBORN/ADULT VARIATIONS	IMPLICATIONS FOR NEWBORN CARE
Respiratory patterns		
Circulatory function		
Hematopoietic characteristics		
Thermogenesis		
Renal function		
Immunologic function		

5. After a long and difficult labor, baby boy James was born with a caput succedaneum and significant molding over the occipital area. Low forceps were used for the birth, resulting in ecchymotic areas on both cheeks. What should the nurse tell the parents about these findings?

6. Mary and Jim are concerned that their baby boy who weighed 8 lb 6 oz at birth now, at 2 days of age, "weighs only 7 lb 14 oz."

   A. How would you respond to their concern?

   B. Describe the procedure you would use to ensure accuracy and safety in weighing a newborn.

7. Susan and Allen are first-time parents of a baby girl. They ask the nurse about their baby's ability to see and hear things around her.

   A. What should the nurse tell them about the sensory capabilities of the healthy full-term neonate?

   B. Name four stimuli that Susan and Allen could provide for their baby that would foster her development.

8. ***Newborn Crossword***

ACROSS:

1. Reflex action produced when a finger is placed in the mouth.
2. Protective mechanism that allows the infant to become accustomed to environmental stimuli.
5. Reflex produced when a light is placed directly in front of the pupil.
7. Space between neonatal skull bones.
9. White facial pimples caused by distended sebaceous glands.
11. Reflex that automatically pushes food out of the mouth when it is placed on the newborn's tongue.
12. Wrinkles/skin folds on the scrotum.
13. Number of veins in the umbilical cord.
14. Intestinal cramps related to a reduction in gastric acidity.
16. Color of diaper stain left by uric acid crystals in urine.
19. Yellowish skin discoloration caused by increased levels of indirect or unconjugated bilirubin.
22. Bluish-black pigmented areas on back and buttocks.
23. Color variation related to vasoconstriction on one side of the body and vasodilatation on the other.
25. Symmetric ______ skin folds of buttocks indicative of proper hip placement.
28. Number of arteries in the umbilical cord.
29. White, cheeselike substance on the skin at birth.
30. Designation for newborns who exceed the size standard for their gestational age.
31. Designation for newborns who fall short of the size standard for their gestational age.
33. When supine arm will extend on the side toward which the head is turned and the opposite arm will flex.
34. Transient, spontaneous motor activity when infant is in an alert state or during episodes of crying.
38. Response of fingers when an object is placed in the palm.
39. Shunt between the two atria is the foramen ______.
40. White, cheesy substance found under the prepuce.
43. Specialized adipose tissue utilized for thermogenesis.
45. Substance that facilitates expansion and stability of alveoli.
46. Flow of heat from body surface to cooler ambient air.
49. Heat loss through vaporization of moisture from the skin.
50. Desquamation present at birth in a postterm neonate.
51. Appearance and disappearance of primitive newborn ____ reflect neurologic integrity.

DOWN:

1. Transient cross-eyed appearance.
3. Total number of blood vessels in the umbilical cord.
4. Startle response to a sudden, intense stimulus.
6. Nares will ______ when respiratory distress is present.
8. Transitory cardiac sound produced by blood flow through the fetal circulatory shunts.
9. Thick, green-black stool passed within 24 hours of birth.
10. Bluish discoloration of hands/feet for first 7 to 10 days.
15. Soft, downy hair on face, shoulders, and back.
17. Accumulation of fluid around the testes.
18. Pinkish areas on upper eyelids, nose, upper lip, back of head, and neck, known as stork bites or ______ nevi.
20. Collection of blood between skull bone and its periosteum as a result of pressure during birth.
21. Small white cyst on gum known as an Epstein's ______.
24. Hyperextension of toes with upward stroke on the sole.
26. Overlapping of cranial bones to facilitate passage of head through birth canal.
27. Red, pinpoint marks most often related to pressure applied to a body area during birth.
32. Turn of head, mouth, and tongue when a hungry newborn is touched on the cheek or corner of the mouth.
35. Designation for newborns who meet the size standard for their gestational age.
36. Method for assessment of newborn at 1 and 5 minutes after birth.
37. Phases of the transition to extrauterine life are termed the first and second periods of ______.
41. Heat loss from body surface to cooler surface in direct contact.
42. Reflex that stimulates peristalsis during a feeding.
44. Erythema ______ is a sudden, transient newborn rash.
47. Lines on the soles of the feet indicative of maturity.
48. A fat or sucking ______ gives each cheek a full appearance and serves to facilitate feeding.

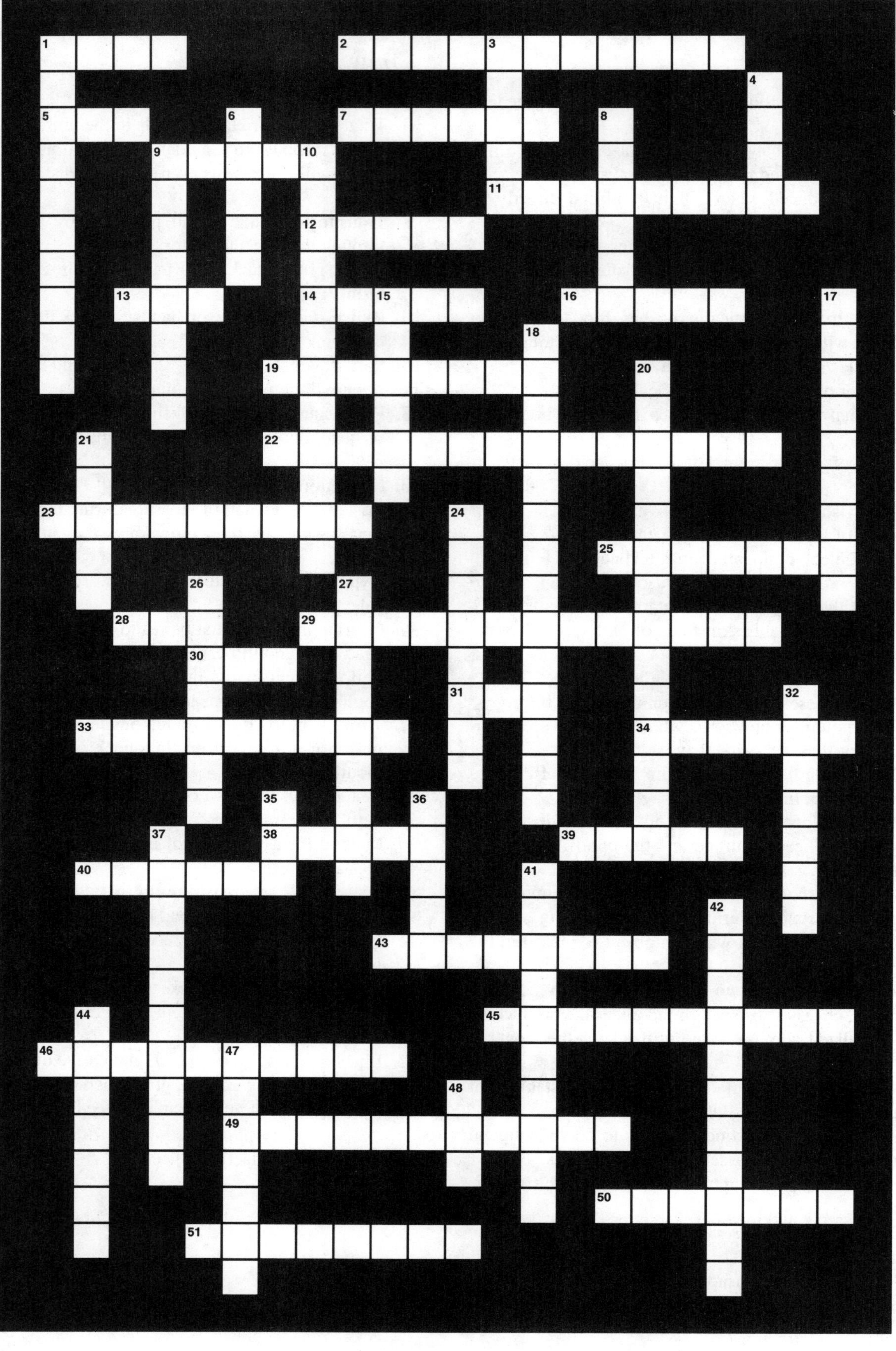

CHAPTER 21 NURSING CARE OF THE NORMAL NEWBORN

1. Apgar scoring is a method of newborn assessment used in the immediate postbirth period, at 1 and 5 minutes. Indicate the Apgar score for each of the following newborns.

   A. Baby boy Smith:
   Heart rate—120
   Respiratory effort—good, crying
   Muscle tone—active movement
   Reflex irritability—cries with stimulus
   Color—body pink, feet and hands blue

   SCORE:______
   INTERPRETATION:
   REQUIRED INTERVENTION:

   B. Baby girl Doe:
   Heart rate—102
   Respiratory effort—slow, irregular
   Muscle tone—some flexion of extremities
   Reflex irritability—grimace with stimulus
   Color—pale

   SCORE: ______
   INTERPRETATION:
   REQUIRED INTERVENTION:

2. Baby boy Jones is 24 hours old. The nurse is preparing to perform a physical examination of this newborn before his discharge.

   A. List the actions the nurse should take to ensure safety and accuracy. Include the rationale for the actions you have identified.
   B. Identify the major points that should be assessed as part of this physical examination.
   C. Support the premise that baby boy Jones' parents should be present during this examination.

3. The newborn must be protected from both cold stress and overheating. For each of the following mechanisms, describe one action the nurse can take to prevent cold stress or overheating:

   Conduction

   Convection

   Radiation

   Evaporation

4. Baby girl Brown has an accumulation of mucus in her nasal passages and mouth, making breathing difficult.

   A. List the steps that the nurse should follow in using a bulb syringe to clear the infant's airway.
   B. If mucus accumulation continues and breathing is compromised, use of a nasopharyngeal catheter with mechanical suction may be required. List the steps the nurse should follow in using this method to clear the newborn's airway.

5. Mary's newborn girl is in a drowsy state when brought to her room to be breast-fed. How could the nurse assist Mary to alter the newborn's state from drowsy to alert?

6. Susan and James are taking their newly circumcised (6 hours post procedure) baby home. This is their first baby, and they express anxiety concerning care of both the circumcision and the umbilical cord. What instructions should the nurse give regarding assessment of both sites and the care measures required to facilitate healing?

7. List the safety and medical aseptic principles that should be followed when sponge bathing a newborn.

8. Andrew and Marion are parents of a newborn who has developed hyperbilirubinemia. They are very concerned about the color of their baby and the need to put the baby under special lights. "A relative was yellow just like our baby and later died of liver cancer!"

   A. Describe how the nurse should respond to Andrew and Marion's concern.
   B. List the precautions and care measures that a nurse should take to prevent injury to the newborn yet maintain the effectiveness of the treatment. Include the rationale for each action identified.

9. Angela, the mother of a newborn, tells the nurse, "I know that I should get my baby immunized, but it is so expensive for each one and there are so many. Since I am breast-feeding, my baby is protected from infection. Do you think it would be all right to wait a while and get fewer injections?" How should the nurse respond?

10. *True or false:* Circle "T" if true or "F" if false for each of the following statements. Correct the false statements.

T F According to the principles of universal precautions, the nurse should wear gloves, gown, and mask when assessing a full-term newborn during the immediate postbirth period.

T F For the first 12 hours after birth, a newborn's temperature should be taken rectally.

T F CPR guidelines for infants recommend cycles of five compressions and one ventilation (a 5:1 ratio), with the five compressions completed at a rate of ≤ 3 seconds.

T F After a feeding, infants should be placed on their left side to facilitate gastric emptying into the small intestine.

T F The recommended site for intramuscular injections in the newborn is the vastus lateralis muscle.

T F A major preventive measure for hyperbilirubinemia is early feeding of the newborn.

T F If bleeding is noted after a circumcision, the nurse should apply gentle yet constant pressure to the site until the physician arrives.

T F To facilitate obtaining a heel-stick blood sample, the loose application of a warm, wet washcloth around the foot for 5 to 10 minutes is sufficient to dilate the blood vessels in the heel.

T F An alcohol swab should be used to apply pressure to the heel after a blood sample is obtained.

T F Before application of a U-bag, the genitalia, perineum, and surrounding skin should be washed, dried, and sprinkled with talcum powder to prevent excoriation.

T F For a single-void specimen, 1 to 2 ml of urine are required.

T F Nonnutritive sucking with a pacifier or finger should be discouraged in the newborn because it leads to malformation of the jaw and to dependency.

CHAPTER 22 NEWBORN NUTRITION AND FEEDING

1. Compute the daily calorie and fluid requirements for each of the following newborns.

INFANT	CALORIES	FLUID
Jim: 1 month, 8 lb 8 oz		
Sue: 4 months, 13 lb 4 oz		
Sam: 7 months, 16 lb 2 oz		

2. Before discharge with her healthy, full-term baby boy, Mary, a primiparous woman, asks the nurse about when she should start solid foods like cereals "so that the baby will sleep through the night." How should the nurse respond to Mary's request for information?

3. Mary Ann is bottle-feeding her baby. She expresses concern to the nurse at the well-baby clinic about heart disease and cholesterol levels as they relate to her 2-month-old baby. She tells the nurse that her family has a history of cardiac disease and hypertension, and she has already changed her diet and wants to do the same for her baby. Mary Ann asks, "When should I start giving my baby skim milk instead of the prepared formula that I am using, which seems to contain quite a bit of fat?" How should the nurse respond to Mary Ann's question?

4. Label the following illustrations as indicated:

   A. *Lactation structures of the female breast*

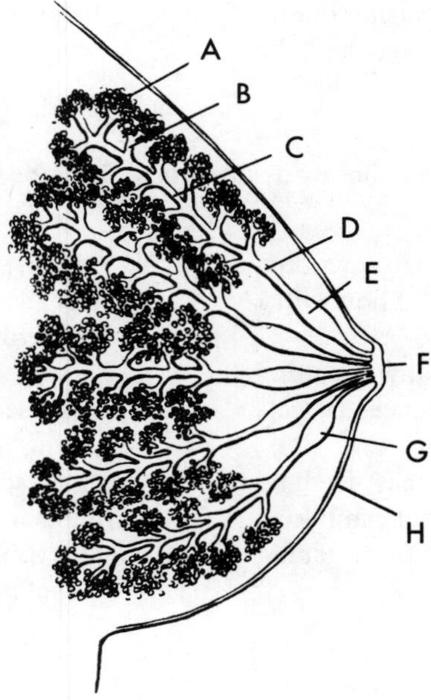

B. *Milk production reflex*

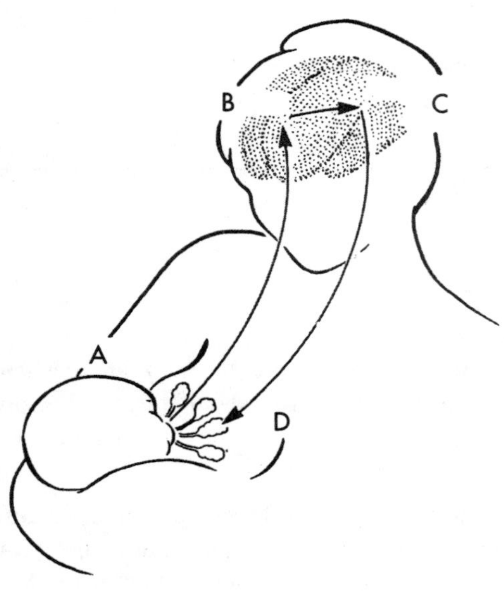

C. *Let-down reflex*

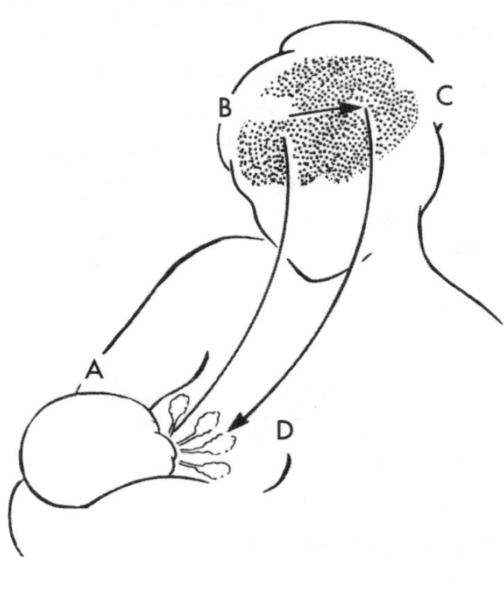

5. Elise and her husband Mark are experiencing their first pregnancy. During one of their prenatal visits, they tell the nurse that they are as yet unsure about the method they want to use for feeding their baby. "Everyone has an opinion—some say breast-feeding is best, yet others tell us that bottle-feeding is more convenient, especially since the father can help. What should we do?"

   A. Why is it important for the pregnant couple to make this decision together?
   B. Why is it preferable to make this decision during the prenatal period rather than waiting until the baby is born?
   C. Describe how the nurse could use the decision-making process to assist Elise and Mark to choose the method that is best for them.

6. Mary, as a first time breast-feeding mother, has many questions. Describe how you would respond to the following questions and comments.

   A. "Everyone keeps talking about this let-down that is supposed to happen. What is it, and how will I know I have it?"
   B. "How can I possibly know if my baby is getting enough if I cannot tell how many ounces he gets with each feeding?"
   C. "It is only the first day that I am breast-feeding, and my nipples already feel sore. What can I do to relieve this soreness and prevent it from getting worse?"
   D. "My friends all told me to watch out for the fourth day and engorgement. What can I do to keep it from happening or at least take care of it when it does?"
   E. "Every time I breast-feed, I get cramps and my flow seems to get heavier. Is there something wrong with me?"
   F. "I am so glad I do not have to worry about getting pregnant again as long as I am breast-feeding. I hate using birth control, and my friend told me I do not have to as long as I am breast-feeding!"

7. Evaluate each of the following actions of Janet, a breast-feeding mother, to determine if the action indicates competency (+) or a need for further instruction (−). For those actions requiring further instruction, indicate what information you would give Janet to correct her action.

   A. Washes her breasts with mild soap and water twice daily. _____
   B. Massages a small amount of breast milk into her nipple and areola after each feeding. _____
   C. Lines each cup of her bra with half a peripad to absorb leakage. _____
   D. Positions the baby on his side and brings her breast toward him, putting the nipple in his mouth. _____
   E. Inserts her finger into the corner of her baby's mouth just before removing him from the breast. _____
   F. Increases her fluid intake enough to quench thirst by drinking water, coffee, juice, milk, and wine. _____
   G. Increases her caloric intake by 500 calories each day with a gradual weight loss noted. _____
   H. Plans to use the "pill" for birth control beginning at 3 weeks postpartum. _____
   I. Wakes the baby every 3 hours at night to feed. _____

8. Alice has decided that for personal and professional reasons, bottle-feeding with a commercially prepared formula is the feeding method that is best for her. She tells the nurse that she hopes she made a good decision for her baby. "I hope she will be well nourished and feel that I love her even though I am bottle feeding."

   A. How should the nurse respond to Alice's concern?

   B. State three principles of bottle-feeding that the nurse should teach Alice to ensure the safety and health of her baby.

CHAPTER 23 POSTPARTUM PHYSIOLOGY

1. Describe how you would respond to each of the following typical questions/concerns of postpartum women.

   A. Mary is a primipara who is breast-feeding. "Why am I experiencing so many painful cramps? I thought this happens only in women who have had babies before."
   B. Susan is being discharged after giving birth 20 hours ago. "For how many days should I be able to feel my uterus to make sure it is firm?"
   C. June is a primipara. "My friend who had a baby last year said she had a flow for 6 weeks. Isn't that a long time to bleed after having a baby?"
   D. Jean is 24 hours postpartum. "I cannot believe it—I look as if I am still pregnant! How can this be?"
   E. Marion is 1 day postpartum. "I perspired so much last night, and I have such large amounts of urine when I go to the bathroom. I hope everything is okay and I can still go home!"

2. True or false: Answer "T" if true or "F" if false. Correct the false statements.

T F After birth, the fundus of the uterus should never rise above the umbilicus.

T F The uterus is slightly larger in size after every pregnancy.

T F Regeneration of the endometrium is completed approximately 6 weeks after birth.

T F Saturating a peripad within 1 hour would be considered a moderate rate of flow for the first 24 hours after childbirth.

T F The external os of the cervix has a jagged, slitlike appearance after a birth has occurred.

T F Until ovulation and menstruation occur, the postpartum woman is likely to experience discomfort during intercourse.

T F The appearance of milk is yellowish and thick compared with colostrum, which appears bluish-white and thin.

T F In most nonlactating women the first menses usually follows an anovulatory cycle.

T F During the first 24 hours after birth an elevated temperature of 100.4°F most likely indicates the dehydrating effects of labor.

T F It is to be expected that the hematocrit and hemoglobin levels will decrease by the third day postpartum.

T F In the postpartum period a leukocytosis of 20,000 strongly indicates uterine or bladder infection.

T F The involution process often produces a mild proteinuria of +1.

3. ***Postpartum Crossword***
(NOTE: Complete after reading both Chapters 23 and 24)

ACROSS:

1. Hormone that stimulates the uterus to contract.
3. Period of postpartum maternal adjustment, indicated by vacillation between a need for nurturing and a desire to take charge.
8. Term used to describe the "fit" between the infant's cues and the parent's response.
9. The interdependent phase of maternal adjustment in which the resumption of the couple relationship is the focus.
10. A method used to check for the presence of a thrombosis by dorsiflexion of the foot.
14. The term used to describe the capacity of the newborn to "dance in tune" to the parent's voice.
16. Surgical incision of the perineum to facilitate birth.
18. Term used to describe the yellowish-white lochia that begins about 10 days after birth.
19. Term used to describe the pink-to-brown lochia that begins about 3 to 4 days after birth.
20. Involution of the uterus that is accomplished by a decrease in size of the ______ cells.
23. The identification of the new baby as a member of the family is called the ______ process.
24. Term used to describe the painful contractions of the uterus that occur after birth.
26. Failure of the placental site to heal completely is called ______ of the placental site.
27. The lactogenic hormone produced in large quantities by the pituitary gland of lactating women.
28. Term used to describe the profuse sweating that occurs during the postpartum period to rid the body of fluid retained during pregnancy.
29. Period of postpartum maternal adjustment characterized by maternal dependency and the need to be nurtured.
30. Term used to describe the distended, firm, tender, and warm breasts of the postpartum woman.

DOWN:

2. Feeling of dizziness or faintness immediately on standing may be attributed to ______ hypotension.
4. Term used to describe the return of the uterus to a nonpregnant state.
5. Separation of the abdominal wall muscles.
6. Term that describes the feeling of affection or loyalty that binds one person to another, as a parent with the newborn.
7. Term used to describe a person's own pattern of activity.
11. Increased production of urine that occurs in the postpartum period, helping to rid the body of fluid retained during pregnancy.
12. Characteristic odor of normal lochia.
13. A type of body movement and behavior that provides the observer with cues to interpret and then to respond.
15. An anal varicosity.
17. Term used interchangeably with postpartum to describe the period of recovery after childbirth.
21. The father's absorption, preoccupation, and interest in his infant.
22. Term used to describe the sloughing off of necrotic tissue as occurs with the shedding of the decidua after birth.
25. The bloody lochial flow that occurs for the first few days after birth.

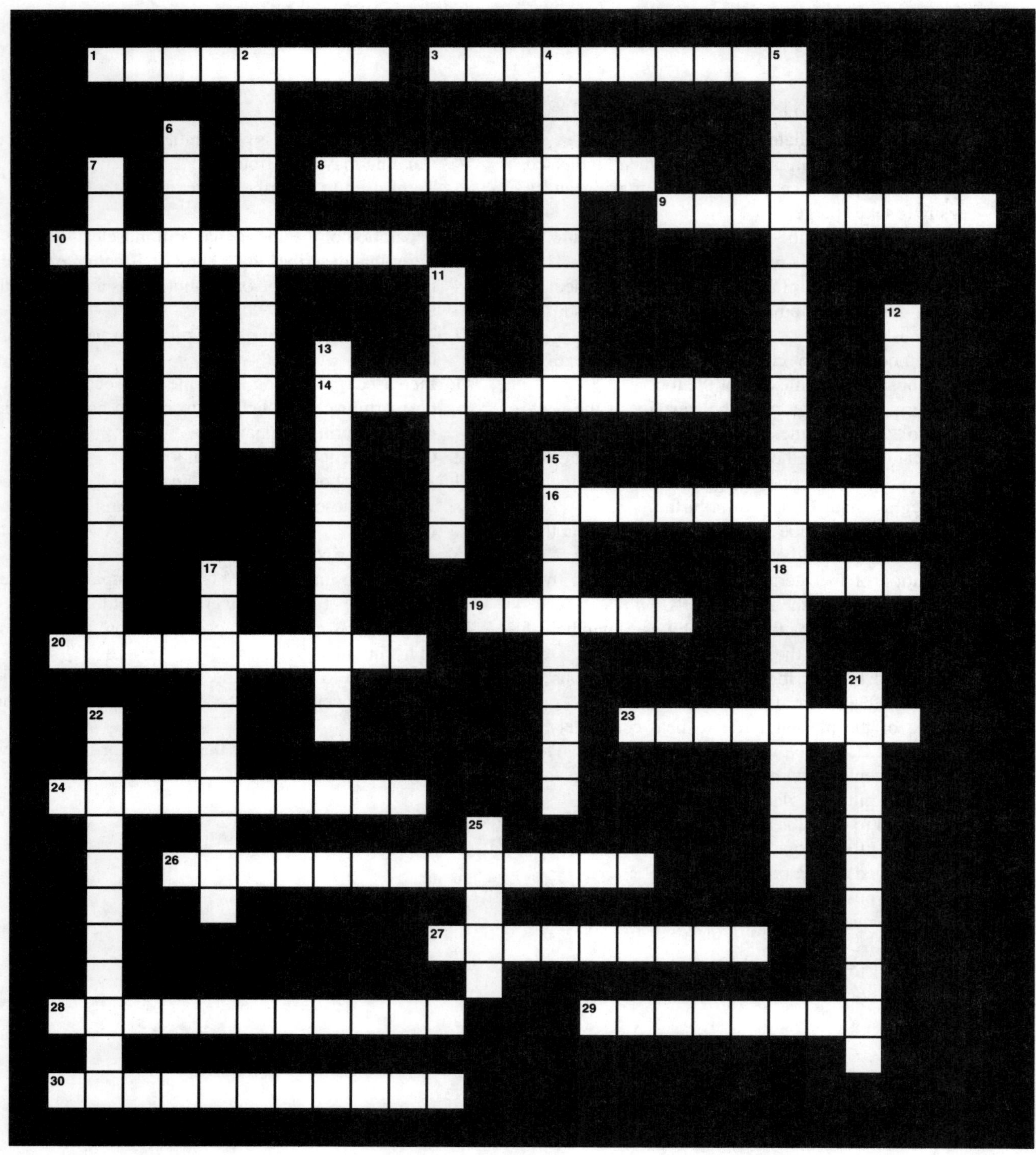

CHAPTER 24 FAMILY DYNAMICS AFTER CHILDBIRTH

1. Jane and Andrew are parents of a newborn girl. Describe what you would teach them regarding the communication process as it relates to their newborn:

   - Techniques they can use to communicate effectively with their newborn
   - The manner in which the baby is able to communicate with them

2. Allison had a difficult labor, which resulted in an emergency cesarean birth under general anesthesia. She did not see her baby until 12 hours after her birth. Allison tells the nurse who brings the baby to her room, "I am so disappointed. I had planned to breast-feed my baby and hold her close, skin to skin, right after her birth just like all the books say. I know that this is so important for our relationship." How should the nurse respond to Allison's concern?

3. Mary and Jim are the parents of three sons. They very much wanted to have a girl this time, but after a long and difficult birth they had another son who weighed 10 pounds. His appearance reflects the difficult birth: occipital molding, caput succedaneum, and forcep marks on each cheek. Mary and Jim express their disappointment not only in the appearance of their son but also in the fact that they had another boy. "This was supposed to be our last child; now we just do not know what we will do." If you were their primary nurse on a SRMC unit, how would you help Mary and Jim bond with their son and reconcile the fantasy of their "dream" child with the reality of their actual child?

4. Angela is the mother of a 1-day-old boy and a 3-year-old girl. As you prepare Angela for discharge, she states, "My little girl just saw her brother. she says she loves him and cannot wait for him to come home. I am so glad that I do not have to worry about any of that sibling rivalry business!" How should you respond to Angela's comments?

5. For each of the following postpartum women, describe the typical behaviors a nurse can expect to see and the nursing measures appropriate to the client's needs and tasks:

CLIENT	TYPICAL BEHAVIORS	NURSING MEASURES
Mary—taking in		
Susan—taking hold		
Alice—letting go		

CHAPTER 25 NURSING CARE DURING THE POSTPARTUM PERIOD

1. Maria has just given birth. Assessment reveals that she and her family are guided by beliefs and practices based on a balance of heat and cold. Describe how you would provide care that is sensitive to her beliefs and practices.

2. Alice is 8 hours postpartum. The duration of her labor was 18 hours. You note that her temperature is 100.2° F.

   A. Identify additional assessment measures required by this finding.

   B. What is the most likely cause for this elevation in temperature at this point in Alice's postpartum recovery?

3. Janice has a midline episiotomy. Describe, step by step, the procedure that you would follow to assess Janice's episiotomy.

4. Judy is 12 hours postpartum and requests medication for pain. Describe the approach that you would take in fulfilling her request.

5. Identify the priority nursing diagnosis, as well as appropriate goals and interventions, for each of the following situations.

   A. Anne is 2 days postpartum. During a home visit the nurse notes that Anne's episiotomy is edematous and slightly reddened. A distinct odor is noted, and there is a build-up of secretions and the Hurricaine gel Anne uses for discomfort. During the interview Anne reveals that she is afraid to wash the area: "I rinse with a little water in my peri-bottle in the morning and again at night. I also apply plenty of my gel."

NURSING DIAGNOSES	GOALS	INTERVENTIONS

   B. Mary gave birth 24 hours ago. She complains of perineal discomfort. "My hemorrhoids and stitches are killing me, but I do not want to take any medication because it will get into my breast milk and hurt my baby."

NURSING DIAGNOSES	GOALS	INTERVENTIONS

   C. Susan, who gave birth 3 days ago, has not had a bowel movement since before labor. She tells the visiting nurse during the interview that she has been avoiding "fiber" foods for fear that the baby will get diarrhea. Her activity level is low. "My family is taking good care of me. I do not have to lift a finger!"

NURSING DIAGNOSES	GOALS	INTERVENTIONS

   D. Martha, a postpartum woman, describes herself as a "failure." Her childbirth experience was not what she expected. "I took medication. I lost control. I know I made a fool out of myself and probably embarrassed my husband. How can I face my Lamaze class friends when they ask me how everything went?"

NURSING DIAGNOSES	GOALS	INTERVENTIONS

   E. Elise and Allan are first-time parents of a 1-day-old newborn. They are observed struggling to diaper their baby. The baby and Judy are crying, and Allan exclaims, "How are we ever going to manage caring for this baby when we get home if we have so much trouble doing such a simple thing that parents should be able to do easily?"

NURSING DIAGNOSES	GOALS	INTERVENTIONS

   F. Agnes is 2 days postpartum. When the nurse makes a home visit, Agnes is found crying. She states, "I have such a let-down feeling. I cannot understand why I feel this way when I should be so happy about the healthy outcome for myself and my baby." Agnes' husband confirms her behavior and expresses confusion as well, stating, "I just do not know how to help her."

NURSING DIAGNOSES	GOALS	INTERVENTIONS

6. *Matching:* Match the description in Column I with the appropriate drug in Column II.

COLUMN I		COLUMN II
A. IV injection of 10 U after birth to stimulate phasic uterine contractions	______.	Methylergonovine (Methergine)
B. Witch hazel pads soothing to episiotomies and hemorrhoids	______.	Oxytocin (Pitocin, Syntocinon)
C. Taken BID for 14 days to suppress lactation	______.	Carboprost (Prostin/ M 15)
D. Oral administration of 0.2 mg q6h during the postpartum period to stimulate rapid, sustained contraction of the uterus	______.	Chlorotrianisene (Tace)
E. Estrogen-containing lactation suppressant	______.	Tucks
F. IM injection of 250 μg to effect rapid, sustained contractions of the uterus within minutes		

7. Anita is a postpartum woman awaiting discharge. Because her rubella titer is 1:6, a rubella vaccination has been ordered before discharge. What should the nurse tell Anita about this vaccination?

8. The physician has written the following order for your postpartum client: "Administer RH_O (D) immune globulin if indicated." What would you do in fulfilling this order?

9. Mary and John express exasperation to the visiting nurse toward their crying 2-week-old baby. "When she cries, we feed her and check her diaper but that does not always work. Friends have warned us about spoiling her if we go to her every time she cries." How should the nurse respond to Mary and John's concerns?

10. Susan, a postpartum woman, confides in the nurse, "My husband and I have always had a very satisfying sex life even when I was pregnant. My sister told me that this will definitely change now that I have had a baby." What should the nurse tell Susan about sexuality after birth?

CHAPTER 26 HOME CARE

1. Early discharge of the postpartum client is a growing trend in the U.S. health care system.
   A. Describe the factors that led to this trend.
   B. State the advantages and disadvantages of this approach to the health care of the postpartum woman.
   C. Mary is in her third trimester of pregnancy. Her physician has suggested early discharge within 24 hours of birth as an option. Mary's insurance company will reimburse her for a 48-hour hospital stay. Faced with this decision, Mary asks you as a nurse for your advice. Describe how you would handle this situation within a nursing process framework.

2. Health teaching is a critical need for postpartum women.
   A. Discuss the constraints and barriers nurses face in preparing and implementing a teaching plan for a woman participating in an early discharge program.
   B. Identify measures nurses could use to overcome the constraints and barriers you identified.

3. Briefly describe each of the postdischarge services that follow. Include the advantages and limitations in your description.

SERVICE	ADVANTAGES	LIMITATIONS
Home visits		
Telephone follow-up		
Warm lines		
Support groups		
Perinatal coaching		

CHAPTER 27 ASSESSMENT FOR RISK FACTORS AND ENVIRONMENTAL HAZARDS

1. *True or false:* Circle "T" if true or "F" if false for each of the following statements. Correct the false statements.

T F The three major causes for maternal mortality are hypertensive disorders, infection, and cardiac failure.

T F Maternal mortality remains a significant problem because a high proportion of deaths are preventable.

T F African-American infants die at twice the rate of white infants.

T F Respiratory distress syndrome continues as the leading cause of infant mortality.

T F A level I facility would be the most appropriate for a woman experiencing normal pregnancy and birth.

T F The major goal of antepartum testing is the prevention of maternal morbidity and mortality.

T F Measurement of the fetal biparietal diameter by means of ultrasonography may be helpful in estimating fetal age and growth.

T F Oligohydramnios, or a decrease in amniotic fluid amount, has been associated with neural tube defects, gastrointestinal obstructions, and multiple fetuses.

T F The nicotine from maternal smoking decreases the resistance in umbilical/uterine artery circulation and affects the systolic/diastolic ratio.

T F The presence of meconium in amniotic fluid antepartally and intrapartally is associated with poor fetal outcome.

T F After amniocentesis or CVS, a woman with Rh negativity should receive RhoGAM.

T F The major disadvantage of a nonstress test relates to its high rate of false-negative results.

2. For each of the following stages of pregnancy, identify three factors that would place the pregnant woman and fetus/neonate at risk:

STAGE	RISK FACTORS
First trimester	
Second trimester	
Third trimester	
Labor	
Postpartum	

3. For each of the following stages, identify five psychosocial perinatal warning indicators for families at high risk for abnormal parenting practices:

CHILDBEARING STAGE	WARNING INDICATORS
Pregnancy	
Labor/birth	
Postpartum	

4. Outline the general process you would follow in preparing pregnant women and their families for antepartal testing.

5. Mary is at 42 weeks' gestation, and her physician has ordered a biophysical profile. She is very upset and tells the nurse, "All my doctor told me is that this test will see if my baby is okay. I do not know what is going to happen and if it will be painful to me or harmful for my baby."

   A. How should the nurse respond to Mary's concerns?

   B. Mary receives a score of 8 for the BPP.

   - What factors were evaluated to obtain this score?
   - What does the score of 8 indicate?

6. *Matching:* Match the antepartal test in Column I with the indication for its use in Column II.

COLUMN I		COLUMN II
A. Biophysical profile	____.	Determination of fetal growth pattern
B. Daily fetal movement count	____.	Estimation of fetal lung maturity based on L/S ratio and presence of PG (phosphatidylglycerol)
C. Ultrasound	____.	Assessment of five factors related to the fetus and its environment
D. Cordocentesis (PUBS)	____.	Measurement of blood flow resistance in umbilical and uterine arteries
E. Amniocentesis	____.	Screen for neural tube defects
F. Chorionic villi sampling	____.	Assessment of fetal condition by maternal monitoring of fetal activity
G. Contraction stress test	____.	Assessment of fetal umbilical blood sample for prenatal diagnosis of inherited blood disorders
H. Doppler ultrasound	____.	Determination of fetal heart rate response to fetal activity
I. Maternal Serum AFP	____.	Assessment for genetic abnormalities conducted during the first trimester
J. Nonstress test	____.	Determination if FHR decelerations will occur with the stress of a uterine contraction

7. Susan, who has diabetes and is in week 36 of pregnancy, has been scheduled for a nonstress test.

   A. Describe how you would prepare Susan for this test.

   B. How would you conduct the test?

   C. Interpret the following tracings. Designate the result each represents, and indicate the criteria you used to determine the result.

   (1)

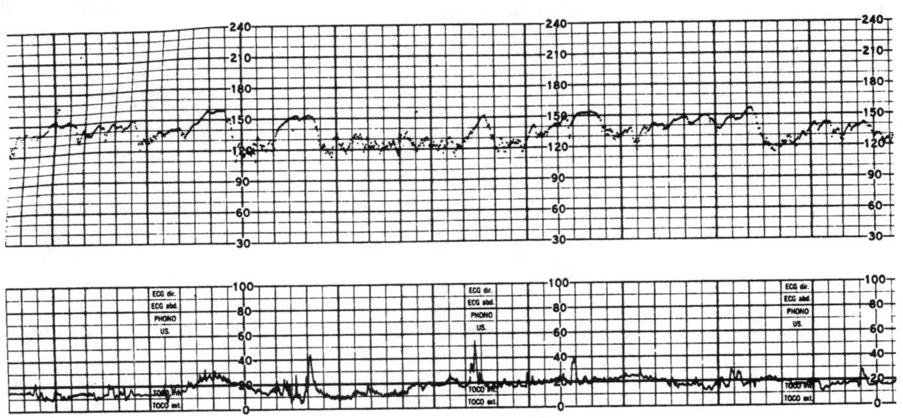

(2)

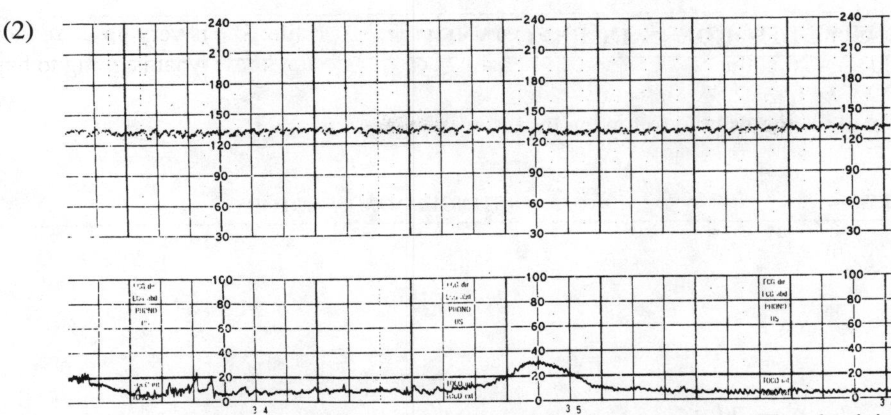

8. Beth arrives for a contraction stress test at the labor unit where you work. The physician has ordered that nipple stimulation should be used to produce the required contractions.

   A. Describe how you would prepare Beth for the test.
   B. How would you conduct the test?
   C. Interpret the following tracings. Designate the result each represents, and indicate the criteria you used to determine the results.

   (1)

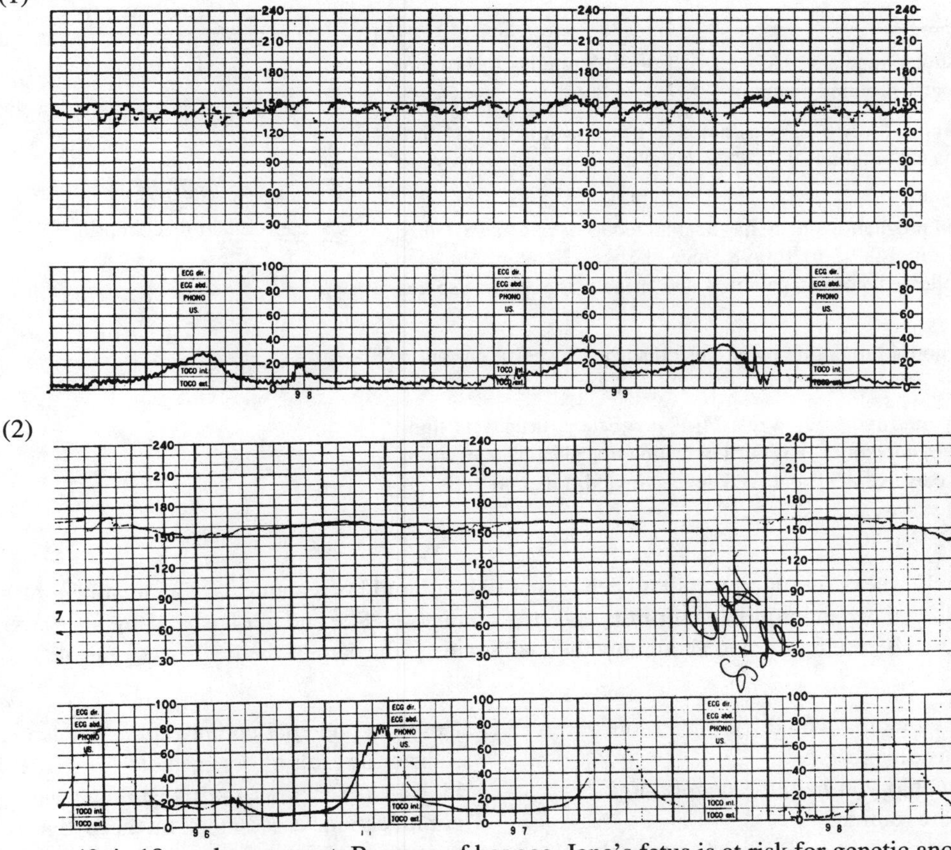

9. Jane, age 42, is 18 weeks pregnant. Because of her age, Jane's fetus is at risk for genetic anomalies, and the physician has suggested an amniocentesis. Identify the nurse's role in the preparation and teaching of Jane with regard to this test.

10. Allison's pregnancy has just been confirmed. As part of the assessment process, a determination of any reproductive health hazards should be made. Outline the approach you would use in making this determination.

CHAPTER 28 HYPERTENSIVE DISORDERS IN PREGNANCY

1. Identify the factors that help to distinguish the following hypertensive diagnoses:

HYPERTENSIVE DIAGNOSES	DISTINGUISHING FACTORS
Gestational hypertension	
Preeclampsia	
Eclampsia	
Chronic hypertension	
Chronic hypertension with superimposed PIH	

2. Contrast the expected physiologic adaptations of pregnancy with the ineffective responses characteristic of PIH:

EXPECTED PHYSIOLOGIC ADAPTATIONS	INEFFECTIVE RESPONSES

3. *Matching:* Match the client description in Column I with the appropriate diagnosis in Column II.

COLUMN I	COLUMN II
A. At 30 weeks' gestation, Angela's MAP ranged from 108 mm Hg to 114 mm Hg; urinalysis indicates protein content of +1.	______. Eclampsia
B. At 24 weeks' gestation, Mary's BP was noted to have risen to 138/84 mm Hg from a prepregnant baseline of 110/66; no other untoward signs were noted.	______. Chronic hypertension
C. Susan, a 34-year-old pregnant woman, has been noted to have a consistently high BP, ranging from 148/92 to 160/98 since she was 28 years old. Her weight gain has followed normal patterns, and urinalysis results also remains normal.	______. Gestational hypertension
D. At 32 weeks' gestation, Maria, with hypertension since 28 weeks' gestation and proteinuria of +3, had a seizure.	______. HELLP syndrome
E. Dawn has been hypertensive since week 24 of pregnancy; urinalysis findings indicate a protein content of +3. Further testing reveals a platelet count of 95,000/mm^3 and elevated AST and ALT levels; in addition, burr cells appear on a peripheral smear.	______. Preeclampsia

4. Jean (2-1-0-0-1) is at 30 weeks' gestation and has been diagnosed with mild preeclampsia. The treatment plan includes home care with bed rest, appropriate nutrition, and stress reduction. She and her husband are very anxious about the diagnosis and also are concerned about how they will manage the care of their active 3-year-old daughter Anne.

   A. What signs and symptoms would have been present to indicate this diagnosis?
   B. As a nurse how would you help the couple organize their home care routine?
   C. What would you teach them with regard to assessment of Jean's status and signs of a possibly advancing condition?
   D. Describe potential complications for Jean and her fetus as a result of her medical diagnosis. Include in your description the physiologic basis for the complication, assessment methods that could be used to detect its occurrence, and measures designed to prevent its occurrence.

POTENTIAL COMPLICATION	PHYSIOLOGIC BASIS	ASSESSMENT METHODS	PREVENTIVE MEASURES

5. Ellen, at 37 weeks' gestation, is admitted to the hospital with a diagnosis of severe preeclampsia.

   A. What signs and symptoms would you expect Ellen to exhibit?

   B. Identify assessment and intervention measures you would institute to protect the safety and well-being of Ellen and her fetus.

ASSESSMENT MEASURES	INTERVENTION MEASURES

   C. Ellen's physician orders magnesium sulfate, 10 g in 500 ml of 5% dextrose in water, to be infused at 2 g/hr. Explain the expected therapeutic effect of magnesium sulfate.

   D. Indicate the most critical assessment measures required to detect the signs of magnesium toxicity:

SIGNS OF TOXICITY	ASSESSMENT MEASURES

   E. What antidote should be on hand before magnesium sulfate therapy is initiated? Look up this antidote in a drug manual to determine its mode of action, dose and route of administration, side effects, and nursing implications as they relate to its use in treating magnesium toxicity.

CHAPTER 29 MATERNAL INFECTIONS

1. Pregnant women are more vulnerable to infection.

   A. State the reasons why pregnant women are more vulnerable to infection.

   B. Describe general measures that can be taught to pregnant women to prevent the occurrence of infection.

2. It is of critical importance that nurses teach women self-assessment and prevention measures with regard to genitourinary infections. List below the typical signs and symptoms that may be discovered with self-assessment for genitourinary infections and the self-care measures that have been proved effective in preventing these infections:

SELF-ASSESSMENT: SIGNS/SYMPTOMS	PREVENTION MEASURES

3. Complete the following table related to infections that can affect pregnancy and its outcome:

INFECTION	MODE OF OF TRANSMISSION	MATERNAL EFFECTS	FETAL AND NEONATAL EFFECTS	TREATMENT MEASURES
Chlamydia				
Gonorrhea				
Syphilis				
Human papillomavirus (HPV)				
Bacterial vaginosis				
Vulvovaginal candidiasis				
Group B streptococci				
Pyelonephritis				
Varicella				

4. TORCH infections can have a devastating effect on fetal/neonatal health status and development. For each of the following descriptions, indicate the TORCH infection it represents:

   A. A viral infection of the liver that is transmitted by droplets or hands improperly washed after defecation ______

   B. Three-day German measles that can produce major congenital anomalies during the first trimester and systemic infection and IUGR after the fourth month ______

   C. A protozoan infection transmitted by consumption of raw meat or improper handling of infected cat litter ______

   D. A viral infection transmitted via contact with body secretions/fluids, including respiratory, genitourinary, breast milk, and blood. It is the most common infectious cause of mental retardation. ______

   E. A viral infection of the liver transmitted in a manner similar to HIV ______

   F. A viral infection transmitted primarily by sexual contact. Active infection of the genital tract at the time of labor requires cesarean birth ______

5. *True or false:* Circle "T" if true or "F" if false for each of the following statements. Correct false statements.

T F The most common STD in the United States today is gonorrhea.

T F Chlamydia can be transmitted only by direct sexual contact or exposure at birth.

T F Gonorrhea can be spread by direct contact with infected lesions and indirectly by transfer from inanimate objects, or fomites.

T F Erythromycin (0.5%) ophthalmic ointment is an effective treatment to prevent infection of the newborn's eyes by both *Chlamydia trachomatis* and *Neisseria gonorrhoeae* organisms.

T F The VDRL result will be positive within 1 week of infection.

T F Even without treatment the chancres from primary syphilis may heal, thus allowing the disease to progress to the next stage.

T F Congenital syphilis can occur throughout pregnancy whenever the spirochetes cross the placenta.

T F It is possible for HIV to be transmitted to the newborn via the breast milk of an infected mother.

T F AZT has been found to be a safe and effective treatment method for women with HIV during pregnancy.

T F Internal monitoring should be avoided in assessing the fetal heart rate patterns during the labor of women with HIV.

T F Determination of a newborn's HIV status cannot be made until approximately 1 year of age.

6. Toxic shock syndrome (TSS) is a potentially life-threatening infection. Identify the three principal clinical manifestations of this infection.

7. HIV infection is increasing among childbearing women.

A. Identify the significant signs/symptoms and psychosocial factors you would include in your assessment of a pregnant woman to obtain information about her HIV risk and status.

B. Indicate the ways in which the HIV virus can be transmitted from mother to fetus/newborn.

C. Identify nursing interventions appropriate in meeting the following goals:

(1) Supporting the immune system of a client with AIDS

(2) Preventing the transmission of the HIV virus while caring for the client during the antepartum, intrapartum, and postpartum periods

8. As a nurse working on a postpartum unit, you must be constantly alert for signs and symptoms of puerperal infection in your clients.

A. What factors can predispose postpartum clients to this type of infection?

B. Identify preventive factors that need to be employed with pregnant and postpartum women.

C. What are the typical signs and symptoms of puerperal infection?

D. What are the critical treatment measures?

E. What are the potential sequelae if the infection is not managed properly?

9. Sara, a breast-feeding mother, begins to exhibit signs and symptoms of mastitis at 2 weeks postpartum.

A. List the typical signs and symptoms of this infection.

B. Identify measures that could have been used to prevent the occurrence of mastitis.

C. Identify the treatment measures and health teaching that Sara needs regarding her infection and breast-feeding.

CHAPTER 30 MATERNAL HEMORRHAGIC DISORDERS

1. Janet is 10 weeks pregnant. She comes to the clinic and states that she has been experiencing slight bleeding with mild cramping for about 4 hours. No tissue has been passed, and pelvic examination reveals that the cervical os is closed.

   A. What is the most likely basis for Janet's signs and symptoms?

   B. What would be the expected medical and nursing management of Janet's problem?

2. Denise, a primigravida, calls the clinic and tells the nurse that she has noted a "good amount of bleeding."

   A. What questions would you ask to obtain a more definitive picture of the bleeding Denise is experiencing?

   B. On the basis of the data collected, Denise is admitted to the hospital for further evaluation. A medical diagnosis of incomplete abortion is made. What nursing diagnosis would take priority at this time?

   C. Identify nursing interventions that would be appropriate for the nursing diagnosis you identified and for the expected medical interventions.

   D. What instructions should Denise receive before her discharge from the hospital?

3. Andrea is admitted to the hospital where a diagnosis of acute ruptured ectopic pregnancy is made.

   A. What findings would most likely be noted during the assessment of Andrea and her status?

INTERVIEW/HISTORY	PHYSICAL EXAMINATION	LABORATORY TESTS

   B. Write a nursing diagnosis that relates to the most critical problem facing Andrea at this time.

   C. Outline the nursing approach you would take related to this nursing diagnosis.

4. Mary has been diagnosed with hydatidiform mole.

   A. Which of Mary's signs and symptoms most typically establish this diagnosis?

   B. After treatment, what must the nurse stress when discussing follow-up management with Mary?

5. Two pregnant women are admitted to the labor unit with vaginal bleeding. Sara is at 29 weeks' gestation and is diagnosed with marginal placenta previa. Jane is at 34 weeks' gestation and is diagnosed with a grade II concealed abruptio placentae.

   A. Compare the clinical picture each of these women is likely to exhibit during assessment.

SARA	JANE

   B. Compare the nursing care required by each of the women as it relates to their diagnosis and to the typical medical management.

SARA	JANE

   C. What considerations must be given top priority after birth for each of these women?

SARA	JANE

6. *Matching:* Match the diagnosis in Column I with the appropriate description in Column II.

COLUMN I	COLUMN II
A. Incompetent cervix	____. Fetus is implanted outside the uterus
B. Abruptio placentae	____. Termination of pregnancy as a result of natural causes before fetal viability
C. Hydatidiform mole	____. Placental implantation in the lower uterine segment
D. Battledore placenta	____. Painless dilatation of the cervical os without uterine contractions, often resulting in the inability to carry the pregnancy to term
E. Ectopic pregnancy	
F. Placenta accreta	____. Trophoblastic cells covering chorionic villi that proliferate and develop into a cystic fluid filled mass
G. Placenta previa	____. Premature detachment of part or all of the placenta from its implantation site
H. Spontaneous abortion	____. Cord insertion at the margin of the placenta
	____. Adherent placenta because of slight penetration of myometrium by trophoblasts

7. Postbirth hemorrhage is a leading cause of maternal mortality.

A Contrast the causative/risk factors for immediate postbirth hemorrhage with the causative/risk factors for delayed postbirth hemorrhage:

IMMEDIATE HEMORRHAGE	DELAYED HEMORRHAGE

B. Identify the nursing measures you would use to prevent postbirth hemorrhage and the assessment techniques you would use for early detection if it occurs.

8. Dana (5-5-0-0-5) gave birth to a 10-pound baby boy after a prolonged labor. Several hours later she began to exhibit signs of mild hemorrhagic shock.

A. Indicate the signs and symptoms most likely exhibited by Dana that would lead to this diagnosis.
B. Indicate the immediate measures that should be taken in this situation.
C. Indicate the ongoing assessments that need to be made to determine effectiveness of therapy and the status of Dana's shock state.

9. Disseminated intravascular coagulation (DIC) can result from a number of obstetric problems.

A. Identify three predisposing conditions.
B. Describe the pathophysiology that leads to DIC.
C. Indicate the clinical manifestations of DIC that would be noted on physical examination and laboratory testing.
D. Describe four priority nursing interventions in caring for the client with DIC.

CHAPTER 31 ENDOCRINE AND METABOLIC DISORDERS IN PREGNANCY

1. Identify and describe the major signs and symptoms of diabetes mellitus and their physiologic basis.

2. *Fill in the blanks:* Provide the missing terms/words in each of the following statements.

   A. The maternal mortality rate for diabetic pregnancies is ____ times higher than for nondiabetic pregnancies.
   B. Diabetes mellitus is a systemic disorder of ____, ____, and ____ metabolism. It is characterized by ____ resulting from inadequate production of ____ or ineffective use of ____ at the cellular level.
   C. Type I is ____-____ diabetes mellitus whereas type II is ____-____ -____ previously known as ____-____ diabetes.
   D. Research has shown that the major factor influencing pregnancy outcome appears to be the degree of maternal ____ ____.
   E. ____ ____ is the term for types I and II diabetes that existed before pregnancy, whereas ____ ____ refers to glucose intolerance first recognized during the pregnancy.
   F. During the first trimester, insulin dosage must be adjusted to avoid ____, but during the second and third trimester the dosage must be adjusted to avoid ____ and ____.
   G. For the pregnancy complicated by diabetes, fetal lung maturation is better predicted by the presence of ____ in the amniotic fluid rather than by the ____ ____.

3. Describe the metabolic changes that occur during pregnancy, and indicate how these changes affect the woman with pregestational diabetes during the first, second, and third trimesters and the postpartum period:

METABOLIC CHANGES IN PREGNANCY	IMPACT ON DIABETES

4. Mary is a 24-year-old woman with diabetes. When Mary informed her gynecologist that she and her husband were trying to get pregnant, she was referred to an endocrinologist for preconception counseling. Mary tells the nurse that she just cannot understand why this is necessary. "I have been a diabetic since I was 12 years old and I have not had many problems. All I want to do is get pregnant!" How should the nurse respond to Mary's comments.

5. Outline the major maternal and fetal/neonatal risks and complications as they relate to diabetic pregnancies. Include the basis for the risks and complications as well as possible prevention measures.

6. Judy's pregnancy has just been confirmed. She also has type I diabetes.

   A. As a result of her high-risk status a variety of additional assessment measures are emphasized during her prenatal period to determine her status and the status of her fetus. Identify these additional measures and their relevance in a diabetic pregnancy.
   B. What stressors might confront Judy and her family as a result of her status as a diabetic woman who is pregnant?
   C. Describe the focus, as well as the required nursing interventions and health teaching required, at each stage of Judy's pregnancy:

	ANTEPARTUM	INTRAPARTUM	POSTPARTUM
Diet			
Glucose monitoring			
Insulin			
Activity			
General care			

7. Elena (2-1-0-0-1) is a 32-year-old Hispanic American woman in week 28 of pregnancy. Elena is obese. Her mother, who is 59 years of age, was recently diagnosed with type II diabetes. Elena's first pregnancy resulted in the birth of a 9-lb 6-oz daughter who is now 2 years old. A 1-hour 50 g glucose tolerance test last week revealed a glucose level of 152 mg/dl. A 3-hour glucose tolerance test was done yesterday with the following results: fasting—108, 1 hr—189, 2 hr—170, 3 hr—150.

   A. What complication of pregnancy is Elena exhibiting? Give the rationale for your answer.
   B. List the risk factors for this condition that are present in Elena's assessment data.
   C. Describe the pathophysiology involved in creating Elena's problem.
   D. Identify the maternal and fetal/neonatal risks and complications that are possible in this situation.
   E. Outline the nursing assessment measures and interventions necessitated by Elena's health problem.
   F. Before discharge after the birth of her second daughter, Elena asks the nurse if the health problem she experienced during this pregnancy will continue now that she has had her baby. She also wonders if it will happen with her next pregnancy since she wants to get pregnant again soon so she can "try for a son." How should the nurse respond to Elena?

8. Jennifer's pregnancy has just been confirmed. She has type II diabetes and is told that she now must learn how to give herself insulin. Jennifer becomes very upset and states, "I cannot possibly give myself a shot. Why not let me continue to take my pills since they have been working fine so far?" Describe how you would respond to Jennifer.

9. Describe how hyperthyroidism and hypothyroidism can affect reproductive well-being and pregnancy.

10. Marie, an 18-year-old primigravida, is diagnosed with hyperemesis gravidarum. She is admitted to the high-risk antepartal unit.

   A. What physiologic and psychosocial factors should the nurse be alert for when assessing Marie following her admission?
   B. Identify two priority nursing diagnoses related to Marie's health problem.
   C. Outline the nursing care measures appropriate for this client.

11. PKU, if undetected in the mother, may have disastrous effects on fetal development.

   A. Indicate the effects maternal PKU can have on fetal development.
   B. Describe how these fetal effects can be prevented.

CHAPTER 32 MEDICAL-SURGICAL PROBLEMS AND TRAUMA

1. Linda, age 26, had rheumatic fever as a child; mitral valve stenosis subsequently developed. She is presently 6 weeks pregnant. This is the first pregnancy for Linda and her husband Sam. As part of her medical regimen, her physician substituted subcutaneous heparin for the oral warfarin sodium (Coumadin) she had been taking before pregnancy.

   A. Linda states, "I cannot give myself a shot! Why can't I just take the medication orally?" How would you respond as to the purpose of this drug and why heparin must be used instead of Coumadin?
   B. What information should the nurse give Linda to ensure safe use of the heparin?
   C. At 3 months Linda's cardiac condition is classified as class II according to the New York Heart Association's functional classification of organic heart disease. The classification class II means _____. On the basis of this classification the therapeutic plan for Linda should include:
   D. In assessing Linda's condition the nurse should be aware of the physiologic and psychosocial factors that could increase the stress placed on Linda's heart. Identify what some of these factors could be:

PHYSIOLOGIC FACTORS	PSYCHOSOCIAL FACTORS

   E. List the symptoms the nurse should teach Linda and her family to look for, which provide indicators of possible cardiac decompensation.
   F. List the objective signs the nurse should look for when assessing Linda's status for signs of cardiac decompensation and heart failure.
   G. The most critical period for cardiac decompensation in the prenatal period is between the ________ and ________ week of gestation because ________.
   H. Indicate the dangers facing the fetus as a result of maternal cardiac problems, especially if decompensation occurs.
   I. Identify four nursing interventions related to the prevention of cardiac decompensation in Linda.
   J. Linda is admitted to the labor and delivery unit. Her condition is still classified as class II. Indicate the rationale for the following interventions used during Linda's labor and birth:

      Emotional support

      Penicillin prophylaxis

      Epidural regional anesthesia

      Left side-lying position for labor

      Birth in the supine position with knees flexed and feet flat on the bed

      Use of dilute IV oxytocin rather than methylergonovine maleate (Methergine) to prevent hemorrhage after birth

   K. Linda should be observed carefully during the postpartum period because cardiac risk continues. Indicate the physiologic events after birth that place Linda at risk for cardiac decompensation.
   L. On the basis of Linda's continuing cardiac risk, what interventions can the nurse use to reduce the stress on Linda's heart during the postpartum period?
   M. Linda indicates that she wishes to breast-feed her infant. How would you respond?
   N. Identify the important factors to consider when preparing Linda's discharge plan.

2. *True or false:* Circle "T" if true or "F" if false for each of the following statements. Correct the statements that are false.

T	F	Folic acid anemia is the most common type of anemia in pregnancy.
T	F	Anemia predisposes the client to postpartum infections.
T	F	A woman in her second trimester whose hemoglobin level is 11.5 g/dL and hematocrit 35% is considered to be anemic.
T	F	A well-balanced diet alone cannot prevent iron deficiency anemia in pregnancy.
T	F	Exacerbations of sickle cell crises are diminished with pregnancy.
T	F	Asthma increases the incidence of abortion and preterm labor.
T	F	Meperidine (Demerol) should not be used to provide analgesia for laboring women with bronchial asthma because it may cause bronchospasm.

T F In pregnancy, ARDS is most likely to be precipitated by pulmonary embolism, DIC, or aspiration pneumonia.

T F In the management of the care of a laboring woman with cystic fibrosis, close monitoring of serum sodium and fluid balance is critical.

T F The pregnant woman is more vulnerable to cholecystitis than is the nonpregnant woman.

T F Symptoms of rheumatoid arthritis subside during pregnancy.

T F Infection is a leading cause of death among clients with systemic lupus erythematosus (SLE).

T F Therapeutic abortion is recommended when a woman has multiple sclerosis because pregnancy can cause irreversible worsening of the condition.

3. Marilyn is a 32-year-old pregnant woman (1-0-0-0-0) who also is paraplegic.

   A. Describe the problems she will face during pregnancy, labor, and birth and the measures that she can use to deal with them.

   B. Because Marilyn cannot push during the second stage, how will birth be accomplished?

   C. Describe the nursing measures of critical importance during the postpartum period.

4. Describe how pregnancy can complicate abdominal surgery.

5. Trauma can occur during pregnancy, especially in the third trimester.

   A. What pregnancy factors can make a woman more vulnerable to injury?

   B. Imagine that you are a nurse working in an emergency room when Alice, an injured pregnant woman at 32 weeks' gestation, arrives by ambulance. The report you receive is that she fell from a two-step ladder while cleaning her kitchen cupboards.

      - What would be your areas of focus during your initial assessment of Alice?
      - How would Alice's pregnancy influence your interpretation of assessment data?
      - Alice will be discharged after evaluation and observation indicate that no major injuries were sustained. As the nurse preparing her for discharge, what instructions would you give Alice?

CHAPTER 33 PSYCHOSOCIAL PROBLEMS

1. Mary, a 35-year old breast-feeding primiparous woman, is beginning her second week postpartum. She and her husband Tom moved from Buffalo, where they lived all their lives, to Los Angeles 2 months ago to take advantage of a career opportunity for Tom. Tom tries to help Mary with the baby, but he has to spend long hours at work to establish his position. When making a home visit, as part of an early discharge program, the nurse identifies that Mary is exhibiting behavior that strongly suggests postpartum blues.

   A. What signs and symptoms did Mary most likely exhibit to lead the nurse to come to this conclusion?
   B. What predisposing factors and behaviors does the nurse need to be alert for that would indicate progression to postpartum depression?
   C. Identify three nursing diagnoses that are relevant to Mary's situation.
   D. Identify measures the nurse could use to help Mary cope with her feelings and the responsibilities that parenting entails.

2. Abuse of and dependence on psychoactive substances has become pandemic.

   A. Describe the general biologic and psychosocial effects that abuse/dependence can have on a woman and her pregnancy.
   B. Describe the factors nurses should consider with regard to each of the following psychoactive substances:

      Alcohol

      Cocaine

      Heroin

      Methamphetamine

      Marijuana

      Phencyclidine (PCP)

   C. What must be considered during the planning and goal-setting stage of the nursing process as it is used with the pregnant woman who is abusing or is dependent on a psychoactive substance(s)?
   D. Identify three nursing interventions for each stage of pregnancy with regard to the pregnant woman who is abusing or is dependent on a psychoactive substance(s):

ANTEPARTUM	INTRAPARTUM	POSTPARTUM

3. *True or false:* Circle "T" if true or "F" if false for each of the following statements. Correct the statements that are false.

T F Social and cultural deprivation is referred to as visible poverty.

T F For economically and socially deprived individuals, preventive health care practices assume a low level of priority.

T F There is a direct relationship between economic status and maternal and infant mortality.

T F Low-income women tend to begin and end their reproductive cycle at a young age because of the close spacing of their pregnancies.

T F Two chief causes for perinatal mortality among poor women are preterm labor and low birth weight.

T F Rejection of the infant is a predominant characteristic of affective disorders.

T F Transient depression (postpartum blues) begins around the second or third day postpartum and can last up to 3 or 4 months.

T F Sleep disorders are common manifestations of withdrawal from psychoactive substance abuse.

T F Abruptio placentae and acute onset of preterm labor are possible outcomes of IV cocaine use.

4. Identify the reasons why an economically deprived pregnant woman may delay entry into prenatal care.

CHAPTER 34 ADOLESCENT SEXUALITY, PREGNANCY, AND PARENTHOOD

1. Adolescents are becoming sexually active earlier and in greater numbers, contributing to the high rate of adolescent pregnancies and sexually transmitted diseases in this country.

   A. What factors contribute to the earlier onset and to the increased number of adolescents who are sexually active?
   B. Discuss the reasons adolescents often give to explain why they avoid the use of contraceptives.
   C. To be effective, what content and approaches must be a part of adolescent sex education classes?
   D. Describe the profile of an adolescent who would be at high risk for pregnancy.

2. How might a pregnant adolescent face the developmental tasks of pregnancy? How would her reactions to each task affect her health practices during pregnancy and the manner in which she cares for her newborn?

   - Accepting the biologic reality of pregnancy
   - Accepting the reality of the unborn child
   - Accepting the reality of parenthood

3. Susan is a 16-year-old mother of a 1-week-old newborn boy. She lives at home with her mother and two brothers. Jim, the 17-year-old father of the baby, would like to have a role in helping with the parenting of the baby but is unsure how he can do this. Home visits by a nurse are part of the discharge plan.

   A. What factors, which can interfere with an adolescent's ability to attain the developmental tasks of parenthood, must the nurse be aware of when helping Susan and Jim attain the role of mother and father?
   B. On the basis of these factors, what approach and measures should the nurse use to establish a trusting relationship with Susan and Jim and to help them develop an effective parenting role?

4. Describe the potential consequences of pregnancy during adolescence:

PHYSIOLOGIC MATERNAL RISK	PHYSIOLOGIC NEONATAL RISK	SOCIOECONOMIC RISKS

   A. What is the twofold role of the nurse aimed at reducing the negative consequences of adolescent pregnancy?

5. Jennifer is a 16-year-old adolescent who became sexually active 6 months ago when she turned 16. She states that she has had a few sexual partners and has come to the planned parenthood clinic for a "check-up" and "the pill—in case I want to use it when I get a steady boyfriend." This will be Jennifer's first experience with a gynecologic examination.

   A. As the nurse assigned to Jennifer, how would you approach Jennifer's assessment to establish a comfortable, trusting rapport with her?
   B. What assessment data must be collected to obtain a full picture of Jennifer and her health?
   C. Identify two nursing diagnoses appropriate for Jennifer.
   D. Discuss two nursing interventions for each of the nursing diagnoses you identified.

6. Anita, a 15 year old, comes to the women's health clinic. She is in tears and tells the nurse, "I think I am pregnant—my period has not come for 2 months now. What am I going to do? My parents will never understand!"

   A. Testing indicates that Anita is pregnant. What points should the nurse emphasize when assessing Anita?

   B. What measures can the nurse use to help Anita cope with the reality of pregnancy and to handle the decision-making process required?

   C. Anita decides to continue the pregnancy and arrange to have her baby adopted. Describe the nursing approaches and interventions that should be used at each stage of Anita's pregnancy:

PRENATAL	LABOR AND BIRTH	POSTPARTUM

CHAPTER 35 LABOR AND BIRTH AT RISK

1. Define each of the following terms related to high-risk labor and birth:

   A. Dystocia
   B. Dysfunctional labor
   C. Precipitous labor
   D. Pelvic and soft tissue dystocia
   E. Cephalopelvic disproportion
   F. Fetal malposition and presentation
   G. Prolonged latent phase
   H. Protracted active phase
   I. Arrested active phase
   J. Protracted descent
   K. Arrested descent
   L. Failure of descent
   M. External cephalic version
   N. Trial of labor
   O. Induction of labor
   O. Augmentation of labor
   Q. Amniotomy
   R. Forceps-assisted birth
   S. Vacuum extraction
   T. VBAC

2. Describe each of the *five factors* that cause labor to be long, difficult, or abnormal, and explain how they interrelate.

3. Angela (1-0-0-0-0) is experiencing hypertonic uterine dysfunction, and Bernice (3-1-0-1-1) is experiencing hypotonic uterine dysfunction. Contrast each woman's labor in terms of precipitating factors, typical signs, symptoms and labor patterns exhibited, and the expected management:

	ANGELA (hypertonic)	BERNICE (hypotonic)
Precipitating factors		
Signs/symptoms/pattern		
Management		

4. Denise, a primigravida, has reached the second stage of her labor with her fetus at zero station and positioned LOP. She did not attend any childbirth classes and is having difficulty pushing effectively. No anesthesia has been used. As a nurse, how would you help Denise use her expulsive forces to facilitate the descent and birth of her baby?

5. A vaginal examination reveals that Marie's fetus is in the RSA position and presentation. What considerations should the nurse keep in mind in providing care for Marie?

6. Angela (2-0-0-1-0) is at 42 weeks' gestation and has been admitted for induction of her labor.

   A. Assessment of Angela at admission included determination of her score on the Bishop scale. What is the purpose of the Bishop scale, and what factors does it evaluate?
   B. Angela's score was 8. Interpret this result in terms of the planned induction of her labor.
   C. Before induction of her labor the physician plans to perform an amniotomy. What are the nursing responsibilities before, during, and after this procedure?
   D. Indicate with a checkmark which of the following actions reflect appropriate care for Angela during the induction of her labor with intravenous oxytocin. If the action is not appropriate, state what the correct action would be.

      (1) ____ Explain to Angela what to expect and techniques used.
      (2) ____ Prepare a primary line with a physiologic electrolyte solution.
      (3) ____ Attach the secondary line of dilute oxytocin (10 U/1000 mL) to the distal port (farthest from the venipuncture site) of the primary IV line.
      (4) ____ Begin infusion at 3 mU/min.
      (5) ____ Increase oxytocin by 1 to 2 mU/min at 30- to 60-min intervals after the initial dose until the desired pattern of contractions is achieved.
      (6) ____ Maintain dose when contractions occur every 3 minutes and last 40 to 60 seconds.
      (7) ____ Maintain or begin to reduce dose once cervix is dilated to 5 or 6 cm.
      (8) ____ Administer meperidine intravenously to Angela through the secondary line containing the oxytocin.
      (9) ____ Discontinue oxytocin drip immediately when a nonreassuring FHR is seen, then notify physician.

   E. Describe the major side effects for which the nurse must be alert when managing Angela's labor.

7. Anne, a primigravida, attended Lamaze classes with her husband Mark. They were looking forward to working together during the labor and birth of their baby. Because of fetal distress an emergency low-segment cesarean birth with a transverse incision was performed after 18 hours of labor. Even though Anne and her son are in stable condition, she expresses a sense of failure because "I could not manage to give birth to my son in the normal way and now I never will!"

   A. What assessment measures are critical when Anne is in the recovery room after the birth?
   B. What are three appropriate nursing diagnoses for Anne's postoperative/postpartum course?
   C. Identify three nursing interventions for each nursing diagnosis.

8. Preterm labor and birth creates significant risks for the newborn.

   A. *Fill in the blanks:*
   Preterm birth is one that occurs after the ______ week but before the end of the __________ week of gestation. Etiologic factors implicated in preterm birth include ____________________, ____________________, ____________________, ____________________, ____________________, and ____________________. However, in approximately two thirds of preterm births the cause is ____________________. Preterm birth is responsible for almost ____________________ of infant deaths. ____________________ agents are drugs that inhibit uterine contractions. An antidote for ritodrine and terbutaline is ____________________, and an antidote for magnesium sulfate is ____________________. ____________________ is a glucocorticoid that can reduce the incidence of respiratory distress syndrome in preterm infants when given at least __________ hours before birth.
   B. Describe the profile of a woman who is vulnerable to the risk of preterm labor and birth.
   C. What health care/life-style measures would you encourage the woman at risk for preterm labor to adopt as a means of preventing its onset?
   D. Identify the signs of preterm labor that you would teach to pregnant women at risk.
   E. What should a woman do if she is at home and she begins to notice early signs of preterm labor such as a contracting uterus?
   F. What are the objective signs a woman in preterm labor would exhibit?

G. Identify the critical nursing assessments and interventions required for safe and effective administration of each of the following medications used to suppress labor:

RITODRINE	TERBUTALINE	MAGNESIUM SULFATE

9. Postterm birth is the birth of an infant beyond the end of week ____ of gestation.

A. Identify maternal risks inherent in postterm labor and birth.

B. Identify the fetal/neonatal risks inherent in postterm pregnancy, labor, and birth.

CHAPTER 36 NURSING CARE OF THE COMPROMISED NEWBORN AND FAMILY

1. Baby boy James has just been born and transferred to the transitional care nursery. A nurse working in this nursery must be alert for signs of respiratory distress.

   A. Describe the progressive signs that would indicate that James is experiencing respiratory distress.

   B. What are the three major nursing measures that would support James' respiratory efforts and help to prevent the occurrence of respiratory distress?

2. Oxygen therapy is a vital component in the care of the newborn experiencing respiratory distress.

   A. What criteria should be used to determine if there is a need for supplemental oxygen?

   B. Describe the purpose and method for pulse oximetry when oxygen therapy is being administered to a newborn.

   C. Identify the indications for each of the following methods of oxygen therapy and the nursing care measures required to ensure their safe and effective administration:

      Hood

      Continuous positive airway pressure

      Mechanical ventilation

3. Anita, a neonate born after 42 weeks' gestation, is admitted to the ICN for observation as a result of the stress experienced during labor and an Apgar score of 6 at 5 minutes. In addition to close observation of respiratory status, Anita must be assessed for and protected from cold stress.

   A. What signs would Anita most likely exhibit if she were experiencing cold stress?

   B. Anita is placed under an overhead radiant heat shield. The nurse attaches a temperature-monitoring thermistor probe to Anita's skin. What are two recommended attachment sites?

   C. Identify five nursing measures designed to prevent or minimize cold stress for Anita while she is in the ICN.

4. Anne, a 3-lb 12-oz (1705 g) preterm newborn at 32 weeks' gestation, is admitted to the ICN after her birth for observation and supportive care. Anne's nutritional needs are a critical concern in her care. Oral formula feedings are attempted first.

   A. What data should the nurse document after each of Anne's feedings to indicate their effectiveness?

   B. What is the acceptable weight loss limit during Anne's first 3 days of life?

   C. The nurse determines that Anne's suck is weak and she becomes too fatigued during oral feedings to obtain sufficient nutrients and fluid. The nurse confers with the neonatologist, and a decision is made to provide intermittent gavage feedings with occasional oral feedings. Describe the procedure the nurse should follow when inserting the gavage tube.

   D. Describe the principles the nurse should follow before, during, and after a gavage feeding to ensure safety and maximum effectiveness.

5. The ICN is a stressful environment for infants and their families.

A. Identify the common sources of stress facing infants and their families in an intensive care environment:

INFANT STRESSORS	FAMILY STRESSORS

B. Nurses working in the ICN must be aware of infant cues and adjust stimuli accordingly. Provide the required information for each of the following:

CUES OF NEONATAL OVERSTIMULATION	SIGNS OF READINESS FOR INTERACTION

MEASURES TO LIMIT SENSORY STIMULATION	MEASURES TO PROVIDE SENSORY STIMULATION

CHAPTER 37 GESTATIONAL AGE AND BIRTH WEIGHT

1. *Fill in the blanks:*

   A. An infant born before completion of 37 weeks' gestation is termed ________________.
   B. An infant born between the beginning of week 38 and the end of week 42 of gestation is termed ________________.
   C. An infant who is born after the completion of week 42 of gestation is termed ______________.
   D. An infant born after 42 weeks of gestation who exhibits the detrimental effects of placental insufficiency is termed ________________.
   E. An infant whose weight is above the 90th percentile is said to be ________________.
   F. An infant whose weight is between the 10th and the 90th percentiles for his or her age is ________________.
   G. An infant whose weight is below the 10th percentile for his or her age is ______________.
   H. The fetus whose rate of growth does not meet expected norms is said to have ______________.
   I. An infant whose birth weight is less than 2500 g is termed ______________. These infants are considered to have had either ______________ or ______________.
   J. Infants weighing more than ______________ and born after ______________ of pregnancy have the best prospect for survival.

2. For each of the following findings, indicate with a "P" if it reflects a preterm infant or with a "T" if it reflects a term infant.

   ____ Pitting edema over the tibia
   ____ Plantar creases on the entire sole of the foot
   ____ No palpable breast tissue
   ____ Slight in-curving of the pinna of the ear; slow recoil
   ____ Smooth, thin skin with visible veins
   ____ Dark red coloring when at rest
   ____ Thinning of lanugo with numerous bald areas
   ____ Testes within rugae-covered scrotum
   ____ Prominent clitoris and labia minora; labia majora does not cover labia minor
   ____ Response to scarf sign—elbow does not reach midline
   ____ Square window—angle of wrist is 45 degrees
   ____ Popliteal angle >90 degrees
   ____ Extension of arms with slight hip and leg flexion

3. The preterm infant is vulnerable to a number of complications related to immaturity of body systems. Indicate the potential problems and their physiologic basis for each of the following:

   - Maintenance of body temperature
   - Maintenance of respiratory function
   - Maintenance of nutritional/glucose balance
   - Resistance to infection
   - Maintenance of renal function
   - Maintenance of hematologic status
   - Responsiveness to parents

4. Mary and Jim are parents of a preterm baby boy.

   A. Parental responses to their preterm newborn progress through several stages. Match Mary and Jim's comments and behaviors in Column I with the stage in Column II.

COLUMN I	COLUMN II
______ Mary says to Jim, "Did you see him yawning?"	A. Stage one
______ Jim is excited, "Did you see how he smiled at me?"	B. Stage two
______ Jim asks the nurse, "What is his temperature today?"	C. Stage three
______ Mary changes her baby's diaper after feeding him.	
______ Mary looks at her baby's face while stroking and touching him.	
______ Mary and Jim tell the nurse that they named their baby James because he "looks just like his Dad as a baby."	

B. What nursing measures should be used to support Mary and Jim and facilitate their progress through the stages and tasks of parenting a preterm infant?

5. Marion's pregnancy appears to be entering week 43.

A. Identify the assessment methods and their findings that can determine if this pregnancy is prolonged and if the fetus/newborn is postterm or postmature.

B. Describe the dangers facing the postmature, the LGA fetus, and the newborn during each of the following stages. Include the physiologic basis for the dangers:

Labor and birth

Postpartum

6. Janet, a pregnant woman at term, is in labor. On the basis of her serial ultrasound findings, her fetus is estimated to be smaller that it should be as a consequence of Janet's heavy smoking during pregnancy and her high-risk status related to mild preeclampsia. Identify the four major complications facing Janet's baby during labor, birth, and the postpartum period. Include the physiologic basis for each potential complication and the signs and symptoms indicative of its presence.

CHAPTER 38 DEVELOPMENTAL PROBLEMS

1. Hyperbilirubinemia results from physiologic and pathologic conditions.

   A. Differentiate the two forms of hyperbilirubinemia as to onset, cause, and treatment. Include the rationale for the treatments identified:

	PHYSIOLOGIC	PATHOLOGIC
Onset		
Cause(s)		
Treatment (include rationale)		

   B. The yellowish discoloration of the skin and other organs is called ____. The deposit of bilirubin on the brain resulting in encephalopathy is called ____.

   C. Explain the physiology of hyperbilirubinemia.

   D. Identify the measures found to be effective in preventing hyperbilirubinemia.

   E. Describe the nursing measures required when a newborn is undergoing phototherapy.

2. Angela, who is Rh negative, had a spontaneous abortion at 13 weeks' gestation, which resulted in what she said was just a heavier than usual menstrual period. Six months later she becomes pregnant again.

   A. An indirect Coombs' test result is positive. What does this indicate?

   B. Is Angela a candidate for RhoGAM? If not, why?

   C. When and to whom is RhoGAM usually given?

   D. Angela's baby is at risk for erythroblastosis fetalis. Briefly describe this condition.

3. Congenital disorders are the leading cause of infant mortality.

   A. Define the meaning of the terms *congenital* and *genetic disorder.*

   B. During the postnatal period the nurse must be alert for signs that a congenital disorder is present. Identify these signs for each of the following systems:

   Neurologic system

   Cardiovascular system

   Respiratory system

   Gastrointestinal system

   Urogenital system

   Musculoskeletal system

4. Briefly describe each of the following congenital disorders.

   Inborn errors of metabolism

   Diaphragmatic hernia

   Tracheoesophageal fistula

   Esophageal atresia

   Omphalocele

   Imperforate anus

   Congenital hip dysplasia

   Exstrophy of the bladder

   Epispadias

   Hydrocephalus

   Anencephaly

   Microcephaly

   Meningomyelocele

   Meningocele

   Talipes equinovarus

   Polydactyly

   Hypospadias

   Ambiguous genitalia

5. Baby girl Jennifer was born with a cleft lip and palate. Describe the support measures the nurse should use to help Jennifer's parents cope with this congenital anomaly.

CHAPTER 39 ACQUIRED PROBLEMS

1. Birth injuries, although decreasing in incidence, are still an important source of neonatal morbidity.

   A. Identify the risk factors that increase fetal vulnerability to injury and trauma at birth.

   B. Describe the signs that indicate a fractured clavicle and the usual approach to treatment.

2. *True or false:* Circle "T" if true or "F" if false for each of the following statements. Correct statements that are false.

   T F A low Apgar score should alert nurses to the possibility that a birth injury occurred.

   T F Cephalhematoma may result in hyperbilirubinemia leading to neonatal jaundice.

   T F Subconjunctival hemorrhage present at birth requires immediate treatment to prevent permanent ocular damage.

   T F Petechiae and ecchymosis will not blanch when digital pressure is applied.

   T F The bone most frequently fractured during the birth process is the femur.

   T F Neonatal spinal cord injuries are almost always a result of a difficult birth from the breech presentation.

   T F Although the mother infected with toxoplasmosis often exhibits no signs and symptoms, there is a 90% chance of transmitting the infection to the fetus.

   T F Maternal infection with syphilis is most dangerous during the first trimester because organogenesis takes place.

   T F Even with adequate treatment the neonate infected with syphilis may experience complications as late as 15 years of age.

   T F Major teratogenic effects of rubella involve the cardiovascular system and cataract formation.

   T F The infant infected with the rubella virus may be a serious source of infection to susceptible persons, particularly pregnant women.

   T F Newborns infected with cytomegalovirus must begin receiving penicillin therapy within 24 hours of birth.

   T F A primary maternal infection with the herpes simplex virus after 32 weeks' gestation presents a greater risk to the fetus/newborn than does a recurrent HSV infection.

   T F Infants born to mothers who drank socially during pregnancy may exhibit fetal alcohol effect (FAE), which could include learning, speech, and behavioral problems.

   T F Maternal heroin use results in a high rate of congenital anomalies.

   T F Marijuana use during pregnancy may result in shortened gestation and precipitous labor.

3. *Fill in the blanks:*

   There has been a(n) ____ in perinatal mortality as a result of diabetic pregnancy over the past 25 years, with the incidence of congenital anomalies still ____ than the general population. During early pregnancy, congenital anomalies are caused by fluctuations in ____ and episodes of ____. Later in pregnancy, maternal forces high levels of ____ to cross the placenta, stimulating the fetal pancreas to secrete increased amounts of ____. This event results in excessive fetal ____, termed ____. In addition, the blood of pregnant diabetic women whose glucose levels are poorly controlled may have a more ____ pH, which adversely affects ____ or ____ exchange. Fetal/neonatal complications can be reduced if maternal ____ levels are maintained within narrow limits of ____ to ____ mg/dL. Poor control is defined as levels greater than ____ mg/dL with ____, ____, or occasional ____.

4. Baby boy Robert, weighing 10 pounds 4 ounces, was born 1 hour ago. His mother has pregestational diabetes. Describe the typical characteristics and signs of complications for which the nurse must be alert in assessing James.

5. Sepsis is one of the most significant causes of neonatal morbidity and mortality.

   A. Describe the modes for infection transmission during each of the listed periods. Indicate the major sites of infection:

PERIOD	MODE OF TRANSMISSION	INFECTION SITES
Prenatal		
Perinatal		
Postnatal		

   B. Identify the risk factors that, if present, should alert the nurse to the increased potential for infection in the neonate.

   C. List the signs a neonate might exhibit that would indicate that infection is present.

   D. Describe two effective nursing measures for each of the following goals:

PREVENTION	CURE	REHABILITATION

6. Baby girl Susan was born 2 hours ago. Her mother tested positive for HBsAg antibodies as a result of infection with HBV. Describe the protocol that should be followed in providing care for Susan.

7. Baby boy Andrew is a full-term newborn who was just born by spontaneous vaginal delivery. Genital herpes recurred in his mother, and her ruptured membranes before the onset of labor.

   A. Identify the four modes of transmission for HSV to the newborn. Indicate the mode most likely to have transmitted the infection to Andrew.
   B. What clinical signs would Andrew exhibit as evidence of an active infection?
   C. Describe the recommended nursing measures related to each of the following:
      (1) Health teaching provided to Andrew's parents
      (2) Health care follow-up for Andrew
      (3) Vidarabine or acyclovir therapy

8. Baby girl Mary is one day old. Her mother's test for HIV is positive.

   A. Discuss Mary's potential for HIV infection.
   B. Mary's cord blood will most likely test ____ for the HIV antibody. Diagnosis of HIV infection could be made when Mary is ____ old.
   C. Name the two infections that, if contracted by Mary, would strongly suggest HIV infection.
   D. Mary's mother wishes to breast-feed Mary because she has read that it can prevent infection. What should the nurse tell Mary's mother?

9. Baby boy Thomas, at 2 days of age, has developed thrush.

   A. Describe the signs most likely exhibited by Thomas that led to this diagnosis.
   B. Name the modes of transmission for this infection.
   C. Discuss the nursing interventions required by Thomas as a result of the characteristics of thrush and the usual medical management.

10. Jane, a newborn, has been diagnosed with fetal alcohol syndrome (FAS) as a result of moderate to sometimes-heavy binge drinking by her mother throughout pregnancy.

   A. What characteristics might Jane exhibit as a result of FAS?
   B. State two nursing diagnoses related to the problems Jane could face as she gets older.
   C. Describe two nursing measures that could be effective in promoting Jane's growth and development.

11. Maternal substance abuse is harmful to fetal and newborn health status, growth, and development.

A. Describe the clinical picture of newborn withdrawal for each of the following substances:

Heroin

Methadone

Cocaine

B. Identify the general nursing measures related to the needs of newborns affected by maternal substance abuse and the typical management of these newborns.

CHAPTER 40 LOSS AND GRIEF

1. Mary, a pregnant woman at 24 weeks' gestation, has been admitted to the labor unit after a prenatal visit at her physician's office. Fetal death is suspected and eventually confirmed. Identify the dimension of mourning represented by each of the comments made by Mary as she responds to her loss.

   A. "The doctor says he cannot find my baby's heart beat but I know you will since you have a monitor here. My baby is okay—I just know it!"
   B. "I know this never would have happened if I had quit my job as a legal secretary. My Mom told me that pregnant women should take it easy. If I had listened I would have a baby in my arms right now!"
   C. "Since my baby died, I just cannot seem to concentrate on even the simplest things at home and at work. I always seem to feel tired and out of sorts."
   D. "It is going to be hard. I will always remember my little baby boy and the day he was supposed to be born. But I know that my husband and I have to go on with our lives."

2. Worden (1991) identified four tasks of mourners. Describe the four tasks and how you would help a grieving family accomplish these tasks as they attempt to cope with the loss of their 4-hour-old newborn girl.

3. Jane (2-1-0-0-1) is a 21-year-old woman admitted with vaginal bleeding at 10 weeks' gestation. She experiences a spontaneous abortion. Jane is accompanied by her husband Tom. Her 5-year-old daughter is at home with her mother.

   A. Describe the approach you would take to develop a plan of individualized support measures for Jane as she and her family cope with their loss.
   B. Discuss three nursing measures you could include in your plan.
   C. At discharge, Jane is crying. She tells you, "I know it must have been something I did wrong this time since my first pregnancy was okay. We wanted to give our daughter a baby brother or sister." Indicate whether the following responses would be therapeutic (T) or nontherapeutic (N). State how you would change the responses determined to be nontherapeutic.

   ______ "You are still young. You will be able to try for another baby very soon."
   ______ "What can I do that would help you?"
   ______ "Do not worry. I am sure you did nothing wrong."
   ______ "It was probably for the best. Fetal loss at this time is usually the result of defective development."
   ______ "You sound like you are blaming yourself for what happened. Let's talk about it."
   ______ "It must be difficult for you and your family."
   ______ "If it had to happen, it is best that it happened this early in the pregnancy before you and your family became attached to the baby."

4. Identify the factors that can influence how a person responds to a loss.

5. Angela gave birth to a stillborn fetus at 38 weeks' gestation. In addition to emotional support, her physical needs must be recognized and met. Considering Angela's loss, identify these physical needs and how you would meet them.

6. Anita gave birth to a baby boy who died shortly thereafter as a result of multiple congenital anomalies, including anencephaly. She and her husband Bill are provided with the opportunity to see their baby.

   A. How should the nurse help Anita and Bill with their decision to see or not see their baby?
   B. Anita and Bill decide to see their baby. How can the nurse make the time spent with their baby as easy as possible and provide an experience that will facilitate the grieving process?

7. Nurses working with families experiencing loss must be able to distinguish normal grieving behaviors from those that indicate complicated bereavement.

   A. Identify those behaviors that characterize complicated bereavement.

   B. Describe the approach a nurse should take if signs of complicated bereavement are noted.

CHAPTER 41 HEALTH PROMOTION AND SCREENING

1. *True or false:* Circle "T" if true or "F" if false for each of the following statements. Correct those statements that are false.

T F The American Cancer Society recommends yearly mammograms beginning at age 38.

T F The aging process and decreasing sensitivity to pain are two factors that interfere with the diagnosis of gynecologic disorders in older women.

T F The American College of Obstetricians and Gynecologists recommend yearly Pap smears for all women.

T F A Pap smear result described as cervical intraepithelial neoplasia (CIN) grade I indicates the presence of cancerous changes in cervical tissue.

T F A woman being treated with hormone replacement therapy for hypogonadotropic amenorrhea is protected from getting pregnant.

T F Primary dysmenorrhea most often is related to excessive estrogen secretion during an anovulatory cycle.

T F The negative signs and symptoms experienced as a part of PMS are related to edema or emotional instability.

T F Endometriosis most likely will develop within 1 year of menarche.

T F Pregnancy is contraindicated for women who have endometriosis.

T F African-American women who are obese have a high probability of developing osteoporosis during the postclimacteric period.

T F The risk for perimenopausal depression and psychosis is low in women who have a high level of self-esteem and value.

T F Hormone replacement therapy using a combination of estrogen and progestin significantly reduces the risk of osteoporosis and cardiovascular disease.

T F Hygienic care is an important focus of care when a pessary is used to hold a displaced uterus in position.

2. Menstrual disorders can affect a woman, her family, and the quality of her life.

A. Identify the risk factors implicated in hypogonadotropic amenorrhea.

B. Mary, a 17-year-old whose menarche began at age 16, comes to the women's health clinic for a routine check-up. She complains to the nurse that her last few periods have been very painful: "I have missed a few days of school because of it. What can I do to reduce the pain that I feel?" Physical examination and testing reveal normal structure and function of the reproductive system. State the nursing diagnosis appropriate for Mary, and identify measures the nurse could recommend to address Mary's problem:

NURSING DIAGNOSIS	RECOMMENDED MEASURES

C. Susan has been diagnosed with PMS. Describe the approach you would take in helping her to deal with this menstrual disorder.

D. Identify the typical signs and symptoms experienced by a woman diagnosed with endometriosis, *and* describe the related pathophysiologic basis for each.

E. Using a nursing drug manual or the PDR, determine the classification, mechanism of action, administration, side effects, contraindications, and nursing considerations for the drugs danazol (Danocrine) and nafarelin, which frequently are used in the treatment of endometriosis.

3. Complete the following table related to the symptoms of the climacterium and postclimacterium.

SYMPTOMS	MANIFESTATIONS	PHYSIOLOGIC/ PSYCHOSOCIAL BASIS	THERAPEUTIC MEASURES
Vasomotor instability			
Emotional disturbances			
Genital atrophy			
Osteoporosis			
Alteration in sexuality			

4. Denise (6-5-0-1-5), a 50-year-old menopausal woman, has been diagnosed with cystocele and rectocele. Describe the signs and symptoms Denise most likely exhibited to lead to this diagnosis.

5. Jane, a 45-year-old slender white woman who works as a secretary, is at the beginning of the premenopausal period of the climacterium. The interview reveals a high intake of fast foods and coffee, along with a smoking habit of one pack per day. She expresses concern about the development of osteoporosis because her mother experienced the stress fractures and dowager's hump characteristic of this disorder and Jane requests information concerning its prevention.

   A. Identify the risk factors for osteoporosis present in this situation.

   B. What advice would you give Jane regarding measures that could be helpful in reducing the likelihood that she will develop osteoporosis and its sequelae?

6. ***Women's Health Crossword***

ACROSS:

3. Disorder characterized by the presence and growth of uterine lining tissue outside the uterus.
4. The alternate dilatation and constriction of blood vessels that lead to hot flushes is termed ________ ____ instability.
5. An abnormal communication between the bladder and the genital tract is called a ____________ fistula.
6. Absence of menstruation.
7. Thinning of the vaginal epithelium as a result of decreasing levels of estrogen is termed genital ______ ______.
9. Test used to examine cervical cells for abnormalities.
11. A complex of signs and symptoms that begins during the luteal phase and ends just before the onset of menses.
14. A gonadotropin-releasing hormone (Gn-RH) agonist administered intranasally or subcutaneously to treat endometriosis.
17. Period of a woman's life when she passes from the reproductive to the nonreproductive stage, with regression of ovarian function.
18. Herniation of anterior rectal wall into the vagina.
19. Androgenic synthetic steroid used as a treatment for endometriosis because it suppresses secretion of FSH and LH.
21. Posterior vaginal hernia.
22. First phase in the transition from the reproductive to the nonreproductive stage of a woman's life.
23. Leakage of urine caused by a sudden increase in intraabdominal pressure, as occurs with sneezing, coughing, and laughing.
24. Age-related reduction in bone mass associated with increased susceptibility to fractures.

DOWN:

1. Painful menstruation.
2. Backward displacement of the uterus with the cervix pointing toward the symphysis pubis.
4. Narrowing or blockage of the passage from the vulva to the cervix.
8. Downward displacement of the uterus.
9. Developmental stage that begins with decreasing fertility and irregular menses and ends 1 year after the last menstrual period.
10. Disordered growth of cells often considered to be precancerous.
12. Painful intercourse.
13. The point at which menstruation ceases.
15. Phase that follows the cessation of menstruation, which is characterized by effects of estrogen deprivation on the genital tract and bones.
16. Abnormal communication between one hollow organ and another or from one hollow organ to the outside.
17. Protrusion of the bladder downward into the vagina.
20. Device inserted into the vagina to support a uterus that is displaced.

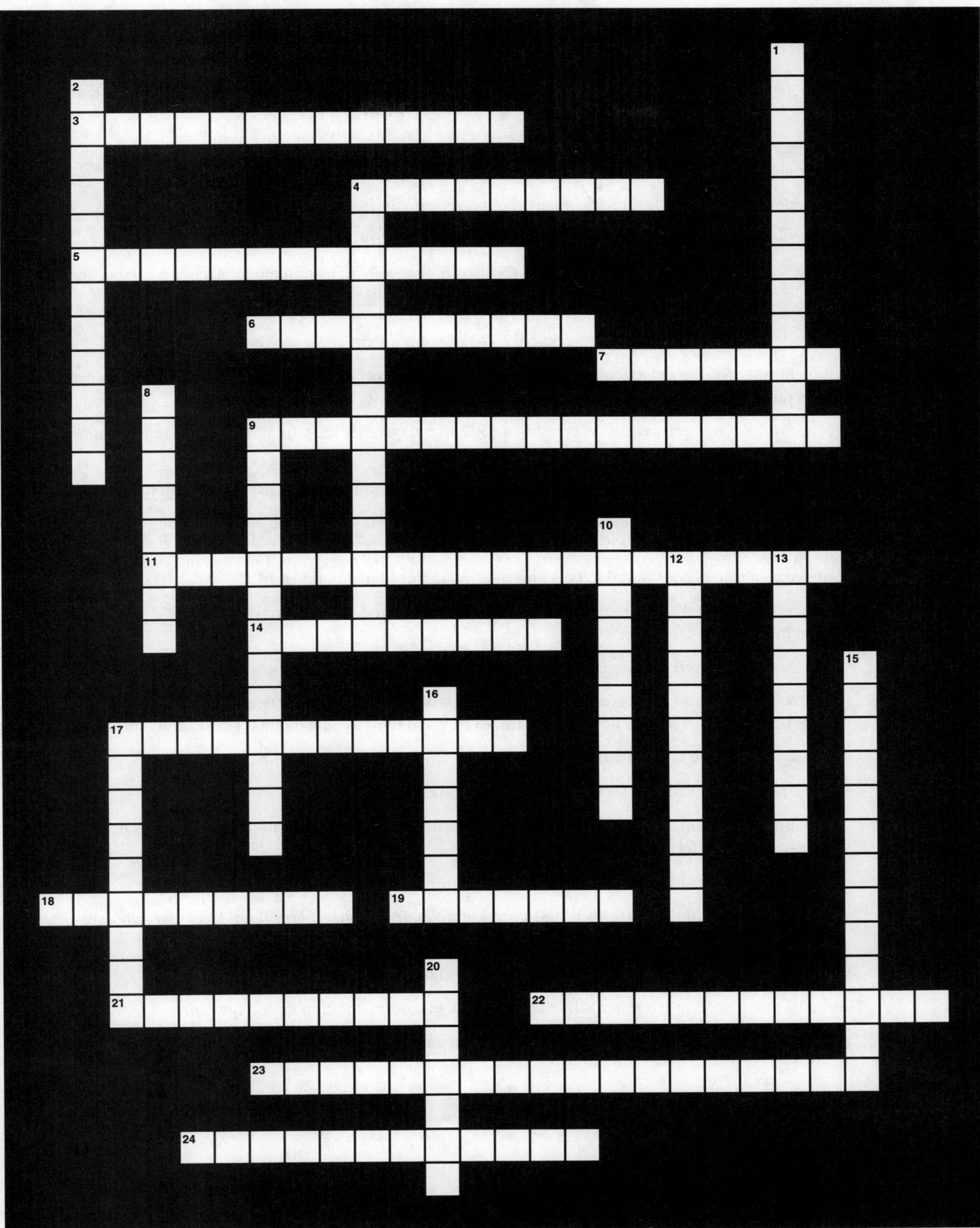
1
2
3
4
5
6
7
8
9
10
11
12
13
14
15
16
17
18
19
20
21
22
23
24

CHAPTER 42 FERTILITY MANAGEMENT

1. *True or false:* Circle"T" if true or "F" if false for each of the following statements. Correct each statement that is false.

T F A contemporary definition of impaired fertility is the inability to conceive or carry to live birth at a time the couple has chosen to do so.

T F Secondary infertility refers to a woman who has repeatedly failed to conceive.

T F As a result of better gynecologic care, the incidence of infertility has decreased.

T F For 80% to 90% of the cases of impaired fertility, a discernible physiologic explanation can be found.

T F Adoption often improves a couple's chance of conceiving.

T F Optimum time for fertilization may be only 24 hours for sperm and 1 to 2 hours for the ovum.

T F Clinical tests for the detection of ovulation such as BBT, cervical mucus, and endometrial changes are based on the secretion of significant amounts of estrogen.

T F Hysterosalpingography, which is scheduled for 2 to 5 days after menstruation, is used to determine tubal patency and to release a blockage if present.

T F Acidity of cervical mucus supports sperm and facilitates their upward transport through the cervix.

T F Use of condoms during genital intercourse for 1 to 2 months will reduce female antibody production in women with elevated antisperm antibody titers.

T F Substance abuse is considered to be a contributing factor in male infertility.

T F Reduction of scrotal temperature by avoiding tight jeans and hot tubs may be effective in treating subfertile men.

T F A history of impaired fertility is considered to be a risk factor for pregnancy.

T F Contraception failure rate refers to the percentage of contraceptive users expected to experience accidental pregnancy during the first year of use, even when they use the method consistently and correctly.

T F The vaginal sponge is as effective for multiparous women as it is for nulliparous women.

T F Use of nonoxynol-9 may offer protection against STDs, including HIV.

T F The Norplant system, which consists of six Silastic capsules containing progestin, provides up to 2 years of contraceptive effectiveness.

T F The most common side effect of Norplant is infection at the implantation site.

T F The IUD is more appropriate than oral contraceptives for women older than 35 of age who are heavy smokers.

T F Voluntary sterilization is the most prevalent method of contraception in the world.

T F In most cases, second-trimester saline abortions require augmentation with oxytocin.

T F RU-486 is an estrogen antagonist that prevents implantation of the zygote.

2. *Matching:* Match the test in Column I with the appropriate description in Column II.

COLUMN I		COLUMN II
A. Laparoscopy	____.	Immunologic test to determine sperm and cervical mucus compatibility and interaction
B. Huhner test	____.	Examination of the lining of the uterus to detect secretory changes and receptivity to implantation
C. Endometrial biopsy	____.	Examination of cervical mucus for sperm motility
D. Hysterosalpingography	____.	Examination of uterine cavity and tubes using radiopaque contrast material instilled through the cervix
E. Sperm immobilization antigen-antibody test	____.	Examination of pelvic structures by inserting a small telescope through an incision in the abdomen

3. Mary and Jim have come for their first visit to the fertility clinic. You must instruct them on the interrelated structures, functions, and processes essential for conception, emphasizing that the couple is a biologic unit of reproduction. Identify and describe each component required for normal fertility.

4. Suzanne has been scheduled for a diagnostic laparoscopy to determine the basis of her infertility.

   A. When in the menstrual cycle should this test be performed?
   B. Describe the preoperative measures required to prepare Suzanne for this procedure.
   C. Suzanne asks you what will be done during the test. What would you tell her?
   D. Describe the postoperative care measures required.
   E. What discharge instructions would you give to Suzanne?

5. With some forms of infertility, pharmacologic measures may be effective. For each of the following medications, indicate classification, mode of action, contraindications, administration, side effects, nursing implications, and content for health teaching. Use the PDR or a nursing drug manual to gather this information:

   - Clomiphene (Clomid, Serophene)
   - Bromocriptine (Parlodel)
   - Human menopausal Gonadotropin (Pergonal)
   - Gonadotropin-releasing hormone

6. Mark and his wife Mary are undergoing testing for impaired fertility. He must provide a specimen of semen for analysis.

   A. What procedure must he follow to ensure accuracy of the test?
   B. State the characteristics that will be assessed and the normal values expected for each.
   C. A postcoital test will be part of the diagnostic process for Mary and Mark. Describe the instructions you would give them to maximize the effectiveness and accuracy of the test.
   D. Identify and discuss four nursing support measures that should be used in working with Mark and Mary.

7. Alternative birth technologies are being developed and perfected, creating a variety of ethical, legal, financial, and psychosocial concerns.

   A. Describe each of the following reproductive alternatives:

      In vitro fertilization and embryo transfer

      Gamete intrafallopian tube transfer (GIFT)

      Zygote intrafallopian transfer (ZIFT)

      Therapeutic intrauterine insemination

   B. Discuss four concerns that are engendered by these alternative technologies.

8. Nora has come to the planned parenthood clinic for information on birth control methods and assistance with making her choice. Discuss the approach the nurse should use to help Nora make an informed decision in choosing contraception that is right for her.

9. June's religious and cultural beliefs prohibit her from using any artificial method of birth control. She is interested in learning about periodic abstinence as a method of contraception. *Fill in the blanks* in each of the following statements concerning this method.

   A. Using the calendar method, June and her husband would abstain from day ________ to ________________ of her menstrual cycle because her shortest cycle was 26 days and the longest cycle was 32 days.

   B. Basal body temperature (BBT) will ________ about ____________ F around the time of ovulation. After ovulation, because of increasing ________ levels, the BBT will ________ about ________ F. This change in BBT will last until __________ before menstruation and is termed the ______ ______. Most authorities recommend abstinence from __________ and for __________ of elevated temperature.

   C. The Billings method would require June to recognize and interpret changes in the characteristics of her ________ ________ such as ______________ and ________.

   D. The symptothermal method combines ________ and ________ with awareness of cycle-phase related symptoms such as ________, ________, ________, ________, or ________.

   E. The predictor test for ovulation detects the sudden surge of ____________ that occurs approximately ____________ hours before ovulation.

10. Alice and Bob use nonprescription chemical and mechanical contraceptive barriers. Label each of the following actions with "C" if correct or "I" if incorrect. For those labeled "I" indicate how the action should be changed.

    ______ When using a spermicidal vaginal foam, Alice applies it immediately before coitus is initiated.

    ______ Alice reapplies the spermicide before each act of intercourse.

    ______ Alice douches within 2 hours of intercourse because she finds the spremicidal foam sticky and uncomfortable.

    ______ When she uses a vaginal sponge, Alice leaves it in place for 6 hours after the last act of intercourse.

    ______ To save money, Alice carefully washes the sponge with water and antibacterial soap and uses it a second time.

    ______ Bob applies a condom over his erect penis leaving an empty space at the tip.

    ______ Bob often lubricates the outside of the condom with Vaseline.

11. Alice plans to use a combination estrogen-progestin oral contraceptive.

 A. Describe the mode of action for this type of contraception.

 B. In the assessment, what factors, if present in Alice's history, would constitute absolute or relative contraindications to its use?

 C. List the side effects that can occur in terms of estrogen excess, progestin excess, and progestin deficiency:

ESTROGEN EXCESS	PROGESTIN EXCESS	PROGESTIN DEFICIENCY

 D. Using the acronym ACHES, identify the signs and symptoms that would require Alice to stop taking the pill and notify her health care provider.

 E. What would you teach Alice about taking the pill to ensure maximum effectiveness?

12. Joyce has chossen the diaphragm as her method of contraception. Label each of the following behaviors with "C" if correct and "I" if incorrect. For those labeled "I" indicate how the behavior should be changed.

 ____ Joyce came to be refitted when she lost 10 pounds as a result of a diet program.

 ____ Joyce inserts the diaphragm a few hours before intercourse to increase spontaneity.

 ____ Joyce applies a spermicide for each act of intercourse.

 ____ Joyce removes the diaphragm within 1 hour of intercourse.

 ____ After removal, Joyce washes the diaphragm with warm water, dries it, and then applies baby powder.

13. Marion has decided to try the cervical cap. What principles should guide her use of this method to maximize effectiveness and to minimize or prevent complications?

14. Anita has just had a Copper-T 380 A IUD inserted. What instructions would you give her before she leaves the office?

15. Judy (6-4-1-1-3) and Allen, both 36 years of age, are contemplating sterilization now that their family is complete. They are seeking counseling regarding this decision.

 A. Describe the approach a nurse should use in helping Judy and Allen make the right decision for them.

 B. They decide that Allen will have a vasectomy. Describe the preoperative and postoperative care and instructions required by Allen.

16. Describe the rights of a client and nurse with regard to abortions, as stated by NAACOG.

17. Edna is a 20-year-old unmarried woman. She is 11 weeks pregnant and is unsure about what to do. She comes to the woman's health clinic and asks for the nurse's help in making her decision, stating, "I just cannot support a baby right now. I am alone and trying to finish my education. What can I do?"

 A. What approach should the nurse use in helping Edna to make the right decision for her?

 B. Edna elects to have an abortion. A uterine aspiration will be performed in the morning. Laminaria will be used as part of the procedure. Edna asks what will happen to her as part of the abortion procedure. What should the nurse tell her?

 C. Identify three nursing diagnoses that apply to Edna and the procedure she is facing.

 D. Describe the nursing measures related to physical care and emotional support that Edna will require as a result of this procedure.

 E. What discharge instructions should Edna receive?

CHAPTER 43 VIOLENCE AGAINST WOMEN

1. Define each of the following as it applies to violence

   Battery

   Sexual assault

   Abuse

   Domestic violence

   Childhood sexual abuse

   Childhood sexual assault

   Incest

   Rape

   Acquaintance rape

   Blitz rape

2. Supply the facts to disprove each of the following myths concerning violence against women.

   A. Spousal abuse is primarily a problem of families who are at a low socioeconomic level and are poorly educated.
   B. Violence affects only a small percentage of women in this country.
   C. Battered women and their abusers cannot change their patterns of behavior.
   D. Battered women often were battered as children.
   E. Battered women usually provoke their attack because they have a need to be beaten.
   F. Women rarely are battered when they are pregnant.

3. Nurses working in women's health care should be aware of the characteristics typical of women who are victims of abuse and the men who abuse them.

   A. Describe the woman who is most vulnerable to battery.
   B. Describe the four types of men who are most likely to become abusive husbands (Elbow, 1977).

4. Research has identified a cyclic nature to battering.

   A. Describe the characteristic behaviors of each of the following phases:

      Phase I: Tension-building state

      Phase II: Acute battering incident

      Phase III: Kindness and contrite, loving behavior

   B. Describe how you could use this information in providing anticipatory guidance for a battered woman who elects to stay with the partner who abuses her.

5. As a nurse working in a woman's health clinic, you must be alert to cues that indicate physical abuse.

   A. Identify the cues you would look for.
   B. Carol, a 24-year-old married woman, comes to the clinic to confirm her belief that she is pregnant. During the assessment phase of the visit, you note cues that lead you to suspect that Carol is being abused by her husband. How would you proceed?
   C. Carol admits that her husband "beats her sometimes and it has been increasing." Now she is afraid it will get worse since she "was not supposed to get pregnant." Discuss the nursing actions that you could take to help Carol.
   D. What would you avoid doing as you work with Carol?
   E. Your effectiveness in assisting Carol depends on your ability to develop a therapeutic/helping relationship with her. Indicate with a check mark which of the following responses will facilitate a positive relationship with Carol.

      ______ "Pregnancy is a stressful time. I notice several bruises on your face. Do you and your husband fight?"

      ______"What kind of person is your husband that he would hurt you and your baby like that?"

      ______"It is important that you leave him now before he hurts the baby as well as you."

      ______"The stresses of a new baby in the family are great. We have a support group in which parents are taught ways to meet these stresses without physical violence. I will ask one of our parent contacts to visit."

6. Susan is an adult survivor of sexual abuse by her father.

   A. What behaviors might suggest to the nurse that Susan is experiencing delayed onset, post-traumatic stress disorder?

   B. What activities could the nurse suggest to Susan that might help her to deal with the past abuse, to heal, and to grow.

7. Marie has been raped. She is admitted to the ER for examination.

   A. Describe the nurse's responsibility in collecting and preserving physical evidence of the rape.
   B. Discuss the nursing actions that should be used to meet the emotional needs of Marie at this time.
   C. Indicate during which phase of the rape trauma syndrome the following manifestations by Marie are likely to have occurred:

      a. Acute phase: disorganization
      b. Long-term phase: adjustment
      c. Long-term phase: integration
      d. Long-term phase: recovery

      ______ Fear of being alone
      ______ Rapid changes in mood
      ______ Anger, humiliation, embarrassment
      ______ Desires to talk about the experience
      ______ Denial and suppression
      ______ Recognizes that integration helped her to grow
      ______ Blames herself for the rape and cites things she "could have done to avoid it"
      ______ Physiologic discomfort
      ______ Initiates self-protection measures by enrolling in a self-defense class
      ______ Physical distress and memories of the rape diminish

CHAPTER 44 NEOPLASIA

1. *Matching:* Match the disorder in Column I with its description in Column II.

COLUMN I	COLUMN II
A. Fibrocystic disease	____. The most common malignancy of the reproductive system
B. Leiomyomas/fibroids	____. Firm, painless, well-defined, mobile breast mass that is unresponsive to dietary changes or hormonal therapy
C. Endometrial cancer	____. Pedunculated tumors usually originating from the lining of the cervical canal
D. Cervical cancer	____. Mammary dysplasia resulting in multiple cyst formation
E. Cancer of the ovary	____. Benign tumors arising in uterine muscle tissue and dependent on ovarian hormones for growth
F. Fibroadenoma	____. Form of cancer that is linked to the human papillomavirus, herpes, and in utero DES exposure
G. Polyps	____. Genital tract cancer with the highest mortality as a result of frequent late-stage diagnosis

2. *True or false:* Circle "T" if true or "F" if false for each of the following statements. Correct the statements that are false.

T F The incidence of mammary dysplasia peaks among women 30 to 50 years of age, with ovarian hormones thought to be a causative factor.

T F The United States has one of the highest rates of breast carcinoma in the world.

T F The risk of an American woman developing breast cancer is 1 in 20.

T F Multiparous, obese, white women are most vulnerable to the development of fibroid tumors of the uterus.

T F The cardinal sign of endometrial cancer is abnormal uterine bleeding.

T F The single most reliable method to detect cervical intraepithelial neoplasia (CIN) is the Pap smear.

T F Preinvasive lesions of the cervix are most effectively treated with internal radiation therapy.

T F The most common symptom of invasive cervical carcinoma is contact bleeding as a result of touch during coitus or physical examination.

T F No visitors are allowed during the course of internal radiation therapy, which lasts about 72 hours.

T F Treatment of ovarian cancer most often requires surgery and multiagent chemotherapy.

T F Cancer is an infrequent occurrence during pregnancy.

T F Pregnancy makes the diagnosis of breast cancer more difficult and may even increase the speed of metastasis.

T F Breast-feeding may continue if breast cancer is detected as long as chemotherapeutic agents are not being used for treatment.

T F Chemotherapy must be avoided as long as a woman is pregnant.

T F Women who have been successfully treated for cancer should wait approximately 2 years before attempting a pregnancy.

3. Mary Anne was diagnosed with fibrocystic breast disease.
   A. What signs and symptoms would Mary Anne most likely have shown?
   B. What measures could the nurse suggest to Mary Anne for lessening the symptoms she experiences?

4. Susan, a 45-year-old woman, was diagnosed with breast cancer in the upper outer quadrant of her left breast. She is admitted for a modified radical mastectomy in the morning.
   A. What risk factors for breast cancer might you note in reviewing Susan's history?
   B. Describe the emotional impact this diagnosis and treatment approach is likely to have on Susan and her family.
   C. On the basis of typical emotional reactions to breast cancer and mastectomy, what nursing measures should be employed to provide Susan and her family with needed support and to facilitate the process of their adjustment?
   D. Identify two priority nursing measures *and* their rationale for each of the following stages in Susan's treatment plan:

PREOPERATIVE	**IMMEDIATE POSTOPERATIVE**	**CONVALESCENT**

   E. What discharge instructions would be important to give to Susan?

5. Marie, age 40, has been diagnosed with two large fibroid tumors.
   A. Describe the clinical manifestations most likely exhibited by Marie.
   B. *Fill in the blanks:*
      Therapeutic management for fibroid tumors depends on ____________ and ____________.
      The three most common therapeutic approaches are ________________, ________________, and ______________.

6. Louise, age 60, has been diagnosed with endometrial cancer. Because of the early stage of the carcinoma, a total abdominal hysterectomy and bilateral salpingo-oophorectomy is the form of treatment choosen.
   A. Describe the nursing care and support required for each of the following stages in Louise's treatment:
   B. What instructions should Louise receive before her discharge?

PREOPERATIVE	**POSTOPERATIVE**	**CONVALESCENT**

7. What are the risk factors that, if present, increase a woman's vulnerability to cervical cancer?

8. Laura has been diagnosed with invasive carcinoma of the cervix and is about to begin a course of radiation therapy.

   A. Complete the following table to summarize the care and support Laura will require at each stage of her treatment regimen.

	INTERNAL RADIATION	EXTERNAL RADIATION
Pretreatment care		
Care during treatment		
Posttreatment care		
Discharge instructions		

   B. Describe three nursing precautions for self-protection during internal radiation therapy.

9. Pat is recovering from a radical vulvectomy as a result of vulvar cancer.

   A. Identify three nursing actions related to the goal: Pat will heal without the development of infection.

   B. Identify three nursing actions related to the goal: Pat will maintain appropriate sexual functioning.

   C. What discharge instructions should Pat receive?

10. Discuss why ovarian cancer is called the "silent" disease.

11. Discuss the issues and feelings that confront a pregnant woman, her family, and her health care providers when a diagnosis of cancer is made.

Answer Key

CHAPTER 1

1. Health focus for perinatal, neonatal, and gynecologic nurses (p. 4).
2. Specific activity to reflect each perinatal/women's health nursing role (pp. 4, 5).
3. Nursing services to reduce potential for neonatal morbidity, mortality, and low birth weight: A variety of answers are acceptable and can be found in the section concerning "Contemporary Issues and Trends." Students can be encouraged to share their ideas in a group discussion (pp. 7–12).
4. F (p. 4), F (p. 8), T (p. 7), T (p. 8), F (p. 8), T (p. 8), F (p. 9), F (p. 9), T, (p. 10), F (p. 8).
5. Problem vs. wellness nursing diagnoses
   - **A.** Characteristics of each (p. 15).
   - **B.** Evaluate nursing diagnoses from clinical experiences: Answers may vary for each student depending on nature of clinical experience. Good basis for postclinical conference discussion.

CHAPTER 2

1. Family structures (pp. 22–24): B, F, H, A, D, G, E, C.
2. Describe conceptual framework: Structural/functional theory (pp. 26–27), developmental theory (pp. 27–28), and interactional theory (p. 28).
3. **A.** ethnocentrism (p. 30), **B.** acculturation (p. 29), **C.** assimilation (p. 30), **D.** subculture (p. 29), **E.** cultural relativism (p. 30).
4. Culturally sensitive communication: Answer should reflect application of content in the section concerning the cultural context of the family (pp. 29, 30), particularly the concept of cultural relativism.
5. Crisis intervention: application to a situation that has crisis potential. Answer should reflect the principles presented in family and crisis (pp. 30–32).
6. ACROSS: **3.** constructive, **5.** socialization, **9.** culture, **11.** relativism, **12.** nuclear, **14.** interactional, **15.** perception, **16.** situational. DOWN: **1.** coping, **2.** economic, **4.** family, **6.** assimilation, **7.** value, **8.** ethnocentrism, **10.** developmental, **13.** maturational.

CHAPTER 3

1. Measures to meet territoriality need (pp. 49, 50).
2. Process in using touch (pp. 46, 49).
3. Characteristics of internal and external locus of control (p. 57).
4. ACROSS: **2.** dysfunctional, **5.** intimate, **7.** neutral, **8.** matriarchal, **11.** acculturation, **13.** past, **16.** present, **17.** future, **18.** efficacious, **19.** ecology, **20.** dialect, **21.** environmental. DOWN: **1.** public, **3.** space, **4.** systems, **6.** external, **9.** transcultural, **10.** roles, **12.** territoriality, **14.** kinesics, **15.** locus of control, **16.** personal, **17.** family.

CHAPTER 4

1. Compare and contrast: Nurse Practice Acts (p. 72), professional standards of care (p. 72–75), and agency policy and procedures (p. 73).
2. Establish/implement process of quality assurance (p. 76).
3. The nursing actions required in the situations described could serve as the basis for classroom discussion. Students can work together with instructor guidance to solve the problems presented. Solutions should reflect application of the ethical and legal principles presented in this chapter, including breech, liability/causation, competency/currency, documentation of care, and the code for nurses.
4. Difference between independent and dependent nursing activities with examples from the text (p. 76) and from clinical experiences.
5. Criteria for documentation (pp. 78–79).
6. Ethical responsibilities of the student nurse: Answers may vary but should reflect application of the code for nurses on p. 80.

CHAPTER 5

1. Establishing a nursing research focus: Apply principles related to use of research in clinical practice (pp. 95–97).
2. Characteristics of quantitative research (p. 88) and qualitative research (p. 88). Each student in a clinical group could complete this assignment. In addition to identifying the factors present in each study that fulfill the requirements for each type of research, the studies could be critiqued using the guidelines presented on p. 96.
3. Role of nursing student with regard to research: consumer of research (p. 95) and use of research in clinical practice (pp. 95–97).

CHAPTER 6

1. *Female Genitalia—External View* Fig. 6–3 (p. 105)
   A. mons pubis, **B.** prepuce of clitoris, **C.** frenulum of clitoris, **D.** labium minus, **E.** skene's duct opening, **F.** Bartholin's duct opening, **G.** vestibule, **H.** fourchette, **I.** posterior commissure, **J.** perineum, **K.** anus, **L.** fossa navicularis, **M.** hymen, **N.** vaginal orifice, **O.** labium majus, **P.** vestibule, **Q.** urethra orifice, **R.** glans of clitoris, **S.** anterior commissure.
   Female Genitalia—Internal View Fig. 6–6 (p. 108)
   A. fundus, **B.** corpus of uterus, **C.** endometrium, **D.** myometrium, **E.** internal os of cervix, **F.** external os of vaginal cervix, **G.** vagina, **H.** fornix of vagina, **I.** endocervical canal, **J.** cardinal ligament, **K.** uterine vessels, **L.** broad ligament, **M.** ovary, **N.** fimbriae, **O.** infundibulum of uterine tube, **P.** ampulla of uterine tube, **Q.** ovarian ligament, **R.** isthmus of uterine tube.
   Female Breast—Sagittal Section Fig. 6–18 (p. 118)
   A. clavicle, **B.** intercostal muscles, **C.** pectoralis major muscle, **D.** alveolus, **E.** ductule, **F.** duct, **G.** lactiferous duct, **H.** lactiferous sinus, **I.** nipple pore, **J.** suspensory ligaments of Copper.
   Female Breast—Anterior Dissection Fig. 6–18 (p. 118) **A.** acini cluster, **B.** milk (lactiferous) ducts, **C.** lactiferous sinus ampulla, **D.** nipple pore, **E.** areola, **F.** Montgomery's tubercle (gland).
   Female pelvis Fig. 6–16 (p. 117) **A.** seventh lumbar vertebra, **B.** sacrum, **C.** acetabulum, **D.** coccyx, **E.** subpubic arch, **F.** ischium, **G.** ischial spine, **H.** pubis, **I.** sacral promontory, **J.** ilium, **K.** iliac crest, **L.** sacroiliac joint.
   Male Genitalia Fig. 6–25 (p. 127) **A.** vas deferens, **B.** urinary bladder, **C.** symphysis pubis, **D.** prostate gland, **E.** urethra, **F.** corpus spongiosum, **G.** corpus cavernosum, **H.** prepuce, **I.** glans, **J.** testis, **K.** scrotum, **L.** epididymis, **M.** bulb of urethra, **N.** duct of bulbourethral gland, **O.** ejaculatory duct, **P.** seminal vesicles.
2. *Menstrual Cycle* Fig. 6–21 (p. 121)
   A. gonadotropin-releasing hormone, **B.** FSH, **C.** LH, **D.** ovum, **E.** follicular phase, **F.** luteal phase, **G.** graafian follicle, **H.** corpus luteum, **I.** estrogen, **J.** progesterone, **K.** menstruation, **L.** proliferative phase, **M.** secretory phase, **N.** ischemic phase, **O.** hypothalamic-pituitary cycle, **P.** ovarian cycle, **Q.** endometrial cycle.
3. **A.** condition of hymen (p. 106); **B.** signs of ovulation (pp. 122–124); **C.** characteristics of female breasts (pp. 117–119); **D.** male sexual development—infancy through childhood (pp. 133–134); **E.** sexual changes with menopause (pp. 124, 138–139); **F.** rubella (pp. 143–144).
4. F (p. 118), F (p. 119), T (p. 120), F (p. 120), F (p. 122), T (p. 124), T (p. 126), F (p. 128), F (p. 133), T (p. 139).
5. Phases of human sexual response: sexual response patterns by Masters and Johnson and Helen Kaplan (pp. 128–131).
6. C (p. 140), E (p. 141), A (p. 139), F (p. 141), D (p. 141), B (p. 140)

CHAPTER 7

1. ACROSS: **2.** XX, **4.** trisomy, **7.** phenotype, **10.** diploid, **11.** monosomy, **12.** gene, **13.** unifactorial, **15.** DNA, **17.** gametes, **19.** meiosis, **21.** heterozygous, **24.** autosomes, **25.** mitosis, **26.** congenital, **27.** enzymes, **28.** oogenesis, **29.** translocation, **30.** spermatogenesis.
   DOWN: **1.** homozygous, **2.** XY, **3.** karyotype, **5.** haploid, **6.** genotype, **8.** teratogens, **9.** mosaicism, **10.** dominant, **14.** recessive, **16.** nondisjunction, **18.** aneuploidy, **20.** chromosomes, **22.** zygote, **23.** gametogenesis.
2. Ovum, ovarian follicle, cilia, tube, 24, sperm, 4–6, 2–3, capacitation, enzymes, ampulla, impenetrable, zona reaction, nuclei, diploid, xygote, 3, morula, blastocyst, implanted, 7–10, decidua, chorionic villi, trophoblasts, basalis (conception, pp. 161–164).
3. Functions of yolk sac (p. 165), amniotic membranes and fluid (p. 165), umbilical cord (p. 167), placenta (pp. 167–170).
4. Fetal circulatory structures: ductus venosus, ductus arteriosus, foramen ovale (p. 170).
5. **A.** description of fetus at 2, 5, and 7 months' gestation (Table 7–1, pp. 180–183); **B.** respiratory function at 35 weeks' gestation and older (p. 171); **C.** quickening (p. 172); **D.** fetal sensory awareness (p. 172); **E.** sex determination (Table 7–1, p. 173); **F.** twinning (pp. 174–176).
6. Answer should reflect understanding of the process of genetic counseling and the nurse's role found on pp. 176–181.

CHAPTER 8

1. Gravidity/parity (pp. 190, 191) **A.** 2-0-1-0-0, **B.** 3-2-0-0-2, **C.** 4-1-1-1-3.
2. 4 (p. 195), 12 (p. 198), 6 (p. 195), 8 (p. 196), 10 (p. 197), 1 (p. 191), 17 (p. 207), 11 (p. 204), 14 (p. 203), 7 (p. 196), 3 (p. 195), 16 (p. 204), 9 (p. 197), 13 (p. 203), 2 (p. 195), 15 (p. 204), 5 (p. 195).
3. **A.** cervical friability (p. 197); **B.** pregnancy testing (pp. 191–192); **C.** increased frequency of vaginal (p. 197) and bladder (p. 202) infections; **D.** breast changes (p. 198); **E.** recommended positions for circulation (pp. 199, 201, 202, 203); **F.** epistaxis (p. 201); **G.** physiologic edema (p. 203); **H.** low back pain/posture (pp. 204–205); **I.** teeth (p. 206).
4. **A.** Alteration in vital signs during pregnancy (pp. 198–202).
   B. 120/76 (MAP 91); 114/64 (MAP 80); 130/80 (MAP 96).
5. Alteration in laboratory tests with pregnancy: CBC (pp. 199, 201); clotting activity (p. 201); acid/base balance (p. 202); urinalysis (p. 203).
6. Alteration in elimination during pregnancy: bladder (p. 202) and bowel (p. 207).

7. Importance of hormones/enzymes increases to maintenance of pregnancy (information found throughout the chapter as the physiologic basis for the adaptations to pregnancy are explained and on pp. 207–208).
   A. parathormone, **B.** insulinase, **C.** estrogen, **D.** progesterone, **E.** thyroxine, **F.** HCG.

CHAPTER 9

1. **A.** weight distribution during pregnancy (pp. 214, 217, Fig. 9–2 [pp. 217, 218]); **B.** pattern of weight gain with appropriate diet (pp. 218, 233); **C.** balanced diet (pp. 219–221, Table 9–1 [pp. 215, 216]); **D.** sodium bicarbonate and pyrosis (pp. 220, 235); **E.** impact of caloric intake and weight gain on fetal development (pp. 214, 218, Table 9–1 [pp. 215–216]).
2. Nutrition counseling for a pregnant Native American woman
   A. Answer should reflect utilization of the steps of the nursing process in creating an individualized plan to meet the client's nutritional needs during pregnancy—nursing process in nutritional care (pp. 221–237).
   B. A variety of answers are possible but must reflect the unique dietary needs of Native Americans as well as the requirements for a healthy pregnancy. Students could also be encouraged to prepare menus for pregnant women representing other ethnic backgrounds (Table 9–1, [pp. 215–216], Table 9–3 [p. 219], Table 9–4 [pp. 224–226]).
3. Importance of and food sources for the major nutrient needs of pregnancy (Table 9–1 [pp. 215, 216]; pp. 218–221).
4. Nutritional planning for a vegan (p. 227).
5. Guidance for a client with lactose intolerance (p. 220).
6. **A.** Goals and interventions for morning sickness (p. 234).
   B. Goals and interventions for knowledge deficit regarding iron supplementation (p. 235).

CHAPTER 10

1. **A.** Manner in which pregnancy is a maturational crisis for the mother (p. 244), father (p. 251), grandparents (p. 255), and siblings (p. 256).
   B. Crisis intervention measures (pp. 50–54).
2. Emotional responses to pregnancy and how the partner can understand and support the pregnant woman: emotional lability (p. 245), view of the partner and his impact on the pregnancy (p. 247), and developmental process during pregnancy (pp. 248–249).
3. Paternal adaptation to and acceptance of pregnancy. Answer should include readiness for pregnancy, concerns and emotional responses, importance of the partner as a necessary support (pp. 251–255).
4. Body image changes and concerns:
   A. Changes and their effect on both pregnant woman and her partner (pp. 245, 247).
   B. A variety of answers are possible here, making this an excellent topic for a group discussion or a focus for a postclinical conference. Students should be encouraged to be creative.
5. Ambivalence during the first trimester (p. 246).
6. Grandparents:
   A. Role of grandparents: mother/daughter (p. 246), father/son (p. 253), grandparent adaptation (pp. 255, 256).
   B. Again, a wide variety of answers are acceptable. Encourage students to see what is available in the community and to interview grandparents for firsthand information on what would be helpful.
7. Father feels "left out of the pregnancy." Review developmental tasks of the mother, especially in the second trimester (pp. 248, 249) and impact of the partner on her pregnancy (p. 247).
8. Impact of pregnancy on sexuality (pp. 247–248). Answer should include how body image (pp. 245–246) can affect sexuality.
9. Developmental tasks of the mother (pp. 248–249) contrasted with the developmental tasks of the father (pp. 251–252).
10. Birth plan, its purpose and how it can be used by the nurse in providing care to the laboring couple: A. purpose (pp. 249, 250, 255); a variety of answers can be given for parts B and C and could serve as a clinical assignment requiring the students to interview nurses and clients regarding the birth plan.
11. Sibling adaptation and preparation (pp. 256–257); sibling preparation box (p. 258).

CHAPTER 11

1. Signs/symptoms of pregnancy (pp. 268, 269) B, A, B, A, D, A, B, A, C, A, C, C, B, D, C, B.
2. Nágele's rule (p. 269) **A.** 2/27/93; **B.** 10/31/92; **C.** 6/15/93.
3. This situation could serve as a basis for group work in terms of addressing problematic clients. Thus a variety of approaches could be taken regarding this client with emphasis on individualizing the approach by using the nursing process and focusing upon the need for the nurse to be nonjudgmental and use therapeutic communication techniques to establish rapport. Components of the interview (pp. 269–272), supportive measures during the physical examination (pp. 272–279), and education for self-care, especially the need for prenatal guidance (pp. 281–287) should be included in the answer.
4. Criteria for BSE (pp. 272–274).
5. Support during the pelvic examination (pp. 274–279) The answer should include not only measures to reduce physical and psychologic discomfort but also health teaching to educate a woman about her reproductive system and how it functions.
6. Specimen collection/laboratory testing (pp. 276–278)
7. Nursing diagnoses, goals, and interventions; nursing diagnoses and goal statements should reflect current professional guidelines.
   A. High risk for urinary tract infection related to lack of knowledge regarding changes in urinary elimination during pregnancy. Interventions (pp. 281–282).

B. Knowledge deficit regarding safe activity during pregnancy. Interventions (p. 285); exercise tips box (p. 286).

8. Cultural beliefs and practices related to pregnancy: describe how they affect prenatal care and identify prescriptions and proscriptions for emotional responses, clothing, physical activity and rest, sexual activity, and dietary practices (pp. 290–292); in addition, student should be referred to Chapter 9.

CHAPTER 12

1. Assessment of emotional well-being (p. 300).

2. Assessment of blood pressure changes and determination of mean arterial pressure should be made for each woman (p. 301); Chapter 8 (p. 199).
Mary: At risk related to increase in BP and MAP 97.
Janice: At risk related to increase in BP.
Susan: Not at risk, related to decrease in diastolic pressure and MAP 84.
Marie: Not at risk, related to decrease in diastolic pressure and MAP 84.
Factors that influence accuracy of BP measurements (Chapter 8, p. 199).

3. Questions of a primigravida during the second trimester.
A. fundal measurement (p. 301).
B. criteria used to determine fetal status (p. 302).
C. alcohol consumption (p. 304).
D. dressing during pregnancy (pp. 304, 307).
E. flatus (Table 12–1, pp. 305, 306). **F.** seat belt (pp. 310, 311).

4. McDonald's rule (p. 301).
16 cm = 18.2 weeks or 4.5 months
20 cm = 22.8 weeks or 5.7 months
24 cm = 27.4 weeks or 6.8 months
Steps to ensure accuracy of measurement (pp. 301–302).

5. Nursing diagnoses, goals, and interventions; nursing diagnoses and goal statements should reflect current professional guidelines.
A. Alteration in comfort related to lower back pain associated with pregnancy at 23 weeks' gestation. Interventions (Table 12–1, pp. 305, 306, and pp. 307–309); Mary's footwear and posture should be taken into account.
B. Anxiety related to previous obstetric losses and lack of knowledge regarding self-care during pregnancy. Interventions should reflect health teaching and counseling that incorporates information regarding assessment of the status of this fetus (p. 302), relaxation/exercise (p. 310), and self-care measures and precautions (pp. 304–313).

CHAPTER 13

1. Normal adaptations to pregnancy during the third trimester: A (p. 326), E (p. 326), F (pp. 324, 329), G (p. 326), I
(p. 326).
Signs/symptoms of potential complications: B (pp. 324, 329), C (pp. 324, 329), H (p. 324), J (pp. 324, 329), K (p. 329).
Warning signs of preterm labor: D (p. 329).

2. T (p. 322), F (p. 323), F (p. 325), T (p. 326), F (p. 326), F (p. 329), F (p. 337), F (p. 331), T (p. 332).

3. Difference between singleton and multifetal pregnancy: answers should reflect a holistic approach that includes the physiologic and psychosocial impact of such a pregnancy as well as the health care and self-care measures required to promote a healthy adjustment (pp. 331, 332, 334).

4. Decision making concerning birth site: answer should include descriptions of each option along with the criteria for use and the advantages and disadvantages of each (pp. 340–344).

5. Pain of childbirth:
A. Potentially harmful effects of pain (p. 337).
B. Nonpharmacologic methods: Gate control (Chapter 15, pp. 374–375); relaxation (p. 338); paced breathing (p. 338); biofeedback (p. 338); therapeutic touch (p. 338); acupressure (p. 338); imagery (p. 339); music (p. 339).

CHAPTER 14

1. *FETAL SKULL* Fig. 14–10 (p. 358); Fig. 14–13 (p. 361) **A.** mentum/chin; **B.** occipitofrontal d. (12 cm); **C.** frontal bone—sinciput; **D.** suboccipitobregmatic d (9.5 cm); **E.** parietal bone—vertex; **F.** occipitomental d. (13.5 cm); **G.** occiput; **H.** sagittal suture; **I.** lambdoidal suture; **J.** posterior fontanelle; **K.** biparietal d. (9.25 cm); **L.** coronal suture; **M.** frontal suture/bone; **N.** bregma—anterior fontanelle.
MATERNAL PELVIS Fig. 14–1 (p. 352); Table 14–1 (p. 354) **A.** anteroposterior d. (≥ 11.5 cm); **B.** coccyx; **C.** transverse d. (≥ 13 cm); **D.** sacrum; **E.** ischial spine; **F.** coccyx; **G.** anteroposterior d. (11.9 cm); **H.** transverse/intertuberous d. (≥ 8 cm); **I.** ischial spine; **J.** sacrum.

2. State presentation, presenting part, position, lie, attitude (pp. 357–360)
A. cephalic, occiput, LOA, longitudinal, flexion
B. cephalic, occiput, LOT, longitudinal, flexion
C. cephalic, occiput, LOP, longitudinal, flexion
D. cephalic, occiput, ROA, longitudinal, flexion
E. cephalic, occiput, ROT, longitudinal, flexion
F. cephalic, occiput, ROP, longitudinal, flexion
G. cephalic, mentum, LMA, longitudinal, extension
H. cephalic, mentum, LMP, longitudinal, extension
I. cephalic, mentum, RMA, longitudinal, extension
J. breech, sacrum, LSA, longitudinal, flexion
K. breech, sacrum, LSP, longitudinal, flexion
L. shoulder, scapula, SCA, transverse, flexion

3. The 5 P's of labor (p. 352): passageway (pp. 352–355); passenger (pp. 355–359); powers (pp. 360–362); position of the mother (pp. 362–363); psychologic response (Chapter 10 and Chapter 13).

4. For each exam the student should describe the position (p. 358), station (p. 361), degree of effacement (p. 362), and dilatation (p. 362) indicated and their meaning in terms of the progress of labor.

5. **A.** Theories as to the onset of labor (p. 364)
B. Premonitory signs of labor (p. 364)

6. ACROSS: **2.** first; **4.** extension; **5.** placental; **7.** ischial spines; **9.** molding; **12.** lightening; **14.** occiput; **16.** presentation; **18.** suboccipito-bregmatic; **20.** attitude; **21.** ripening; **22.** posterior; **24.** bregma; **25.** efface; **27.** prodromal; **30.** pushing; **31.** bony pelvis; **33.** lie; **34.** internal; **35.** frequency; **36.** dilate; **37.** intensity; **38.** duration.
DOWN: **1.** external; **3.** second; **6.** bloody; **8.** station; **9.** mentum; **10.** fourth; **11.** cephalic; **13.** gynecoid; **15.** partogram; **17.** restitution; **19.** sacrum; **22.** primary powers; **23.** breech; **26.** flexion; **27.** position; **28.** sagittal; **29.** descent; **32.** engaged.

CHAPTER 15

1. Physical basis for labor pain (p. 374).
2. **A.** Physical signs and affective expressions of labor pain (p. 374).
   B. Measures to alter perception of pain: student should utilize theory related to pain perception (pp. 374–375) including culture, fatigue, gate control, etc., in determining nursing interventions.
3. Client's unrealistic expectations related to prelabor preparation and anticipated effect on labor pain; student should include information regarding basis for pain (p. 374), nursing interventions related to client support and options available for pain relief (p. 389).
4. Table related to pharmacologic methods, their effects, criteria for use, and nursing management required: systemics (p. 377–378); nerve blocks (pp. 378–386); general anesthetics (pp. 386–387).

CHAPTER 16

1. **A.** Factors associated with a reduction in fetal oxygen supply (p. 398).
   B. Characteristics of a reassuring FHR pattern (pp. 398, 399).
   C. Characteristics of normal uterine activity (p. 398).
2. Nursing support required by maternal anxiety and knowledge deficit concerning electronic fetal monitoring; box: care of mother undergoing fetal monitoring (p. 415).
3. **A.** Late deceleration, Table 16–5, (p. 408).
   B. Nursing actions: answer should include alteration in maternal position and intrauterine resuscitation measures, Table 16–5 (p. 409 and p. 412).
4. Preventive measures: discouraging Valsalva maneuver, maternal position changes, assistance with breathing techniques (pp. 411, 412).
5. H (p. 401); E (p. 399); F (p. 399); G (p. 398); B (p. 403); A (p. 406); C (p. 408); D (p. 408).
6. Table presenting the advantages as well as the disadvantages/limitations for: periodic auscultation (p. 399), external monitoring (p. 400), and internal monitoring (p. 401).
7. Interpretation of monitor tracings: student should include analysis of FHR pattern (p. 411) for variability (p. 403), baseline rate (p. 401), and evidence of periodic changes (p. 403) as well as analysis of uterine activity (p. 398).
   A. Normal, reassuring FHR pattern and uterine activity (pp. 398–399).
   B. Late decelerations, Table 16–5 (p. 408).
   C. Bradycardia, Table 16–2 (p. 402).
   D. Early decelerations, Table 16–4 (p. 406).
   E. Accelerations with uterine contractions, Fig. 16–6 (p. 404); Table 16–4 (p. 406).
   F. Fetal tachycardia Table 16–2 (p. 402).
   G. Mild variable decelerations Table 16–5 (p. 408).
   H. Severe variable decelerations, Table 16–5 (p. 408).

CHAPTER 17

1. Distinguishing true from false labor (p. 425) **A.** 1; **B.** 2; **C.** 2; **D.** 1; **E.** 1; **F.** 2; **G.** 1; **H.** 2; **I.** 1; **J.** 1.
2. Focus of the answer should be the determination of the status of the woman and her labor. Incorporate principles of the telephone interview (p. 425) and data to include in the interview (pp. 427–428).
3. Data to gather from the prenatal record of a multigravid woman (p. 427).
4. Psychosocial support measures for women at varying stages of labor, Table 17–5 (p. 454; pp. 452–458). Susan: active phase; Alice: transition phase; Debra: latent phase.
5. Placement of external fetal monitor: determine location of PMI (p. 433) using Leopold's maneuvers (pp. 437, 438, 439).
6. **A.** Purpose of vaginal examinations (p. 437); answer should also include a description of the information obtained by the monitor (Chapter 16).
   B. Procedure to follow when performing a vaginal examination (p. 441).
7. Diagram of uterine contractions: should be labeled as Fig. 17–5 (p. 434). Method used to assess uterine contractions using the palpation method (pp. 433–435).
8. **A.** Prioritized actions following membrane rupture: FHR (p. 441), vaginal examination to assess for prolapse and condition of cervix (pp. 449–450) and assessment of fluid (pp. 441–442).
   B. Immediate care for protruding, prolapsed cord (pp. 450–452).
9. Anxiety related to lack of knowledge and experience with regard to the process of childbirth. Interventions should include support measures (pp. 452–460) and reflect support of both partners. Goals identified should be realistic, measurable client behaviors.

CHAPTER 18

1. Advantages of new approaches to childbirth: listening to her body (p. 470), maternal position (p. 473), bearing down efforts (p. 473) and birthing beds/chairs (p. 474).
2. F (pp. 470, 472, 473); T (p. 470); F (pp. 472, 474); F (p. 471); T (p. 471); T (p. 473); T (p. 472); F (p. 479); T (p. 482); F (p. 485); T (p. 494); F (493); T (p. 496); T (p. 496).
3. Second stage of labor: events, behavior, and support measures for the latent/resting phase, descent phase, and the final/transition phase, Table 18–2 (p. 475).
4. Immediate measures to prevent maternal hemorrhage following home birth (p. 485).

5. Third stage of labor:
   A. Mechanism of placental separation (p. 486, Fig. 18–11 [p. 489]).
   B. Signs indicative of separation (p. 488).
   C. Measures to assist with placental expulsion (p. 490).
6. Immediate newborn assessment/care following birth:
   A. Five priority assessments related to physiologic integrity (p. 493).
   B. Measures to promote physiologic integrity (p. 494, Table 18–4 [p. 495]).
   C. Measures to foster parent-newborn attachment (p. 491).

CHAPTER 19

1. Care of woman: 4th stage of labor
   A. Importance of fundal assessment: answer must not only include factual information but also reflect concern for and acknowledgment of the client's feelings (p. 507).
   B. Technique of fundal assessment (p. 507, Fig. 19–1).
   C. Fundal characteristics (p. 507).
   D. Timing and method for fundal message (p. 507).
2. Influence of bladder distention upon fundus (p. 507).
3. Examination of episiotomy (p. 508).
   A. Recommended maternal position for examination.
   B. REEDA system.
4. Fundal elevation and deviation from midline (p. 507).
   A. Bladder distention.
   B. Empty bladder through voiding if possible or, if not, catheterization.
5. Safety measures related to assisting postpartum client OOB for the first time: answer should include assessment data that should be gathered concerning the client's current status, circumstances during labor and birth, effect of orthostatic hypotension, access to ammonia capsules, assistance with ambulation, and notation of client's reactions to activity) (p. 511).
6. Criteria to be met before providing newly delivered woman with oral fluids/food: answer should include type of anesthesia as well as current condition with consideration of potential for emergency care that would require general anesthesia (pp. 512, 513).
7. Maternal disinterest in newborn during 4th stage of labor:
   A. Possible rationale for behavior: answer should include recognition of maternal physical status as well as psychosocial and cultural factors (pp. 513–514).
   B. Nursing measures to encourage maternal newborn interaction (p. 514).
8. Contrast expected signs/symptoms of 4th stage of labor with those suggestive of hypovolemic shock: answer should consider degree of bleeding, vital signs, appearance, behavior, and subjective "feelings" (pp. 509, 510).
9. C (p. 506), F (p. 506), E (p. 506), G (p. 508), H (p. 511), A (p. 506, 508), B (p. 511), D (p. 508).

CHAPTER 20

1. **A.** P (pp. 527, 560); **B.** N (pp. 527, 560); **C.** N (pp. 527, 560); **D.** N (pp. 539, 561); **E.** P (pp. 538, 561); **F.** N (p. 535); **G.** P (pp. 528, 560); **H.** P (pp. 554, 561); **I.** N (pp. 530. 559); **J.** N (p. 543); **K.** P (p. 531); **L.** N (pp. 537, 558, 566); **M.** P (pp. 543, 544, 558, 568); **N.** N (pp. 555, 563); **O.** N (pp. 542, 567).
2. Interrelationship of respiratory function (pp. 527, 528), cardiovascular function (pp. 528–532), and thermogenesis (pp. 532–534).
3. Behavioral states/characteristics (pp. 569–571): sleep–wake; 2; 4; quiet alert; active alert; 17; deep; light.
4. Difference in physiologic functioning on newborn and adult level with implications for newborn care related to: respiratory patterns (p. 527), circulatory function (p. 528), hematopoietic characteristics (p. 531), thermogenesis (p. 532), renal function (p. 534), and immunologic function (p. 539).
5. Basis for cephalhematoma (p. 540, Fig. 20–68) and molding (p. 543) with ecchymotic areas (p. 541) on each cheek following a forceps delivery: answer should include an explanation of the findings and prognosis as well as reflect concern for the feelings of the parents.
6. Parental concern regarding weight loss (p. 553).
   A. Weight loss is 8 oz. of 6% of birth weight: finding is within normal limits of 5% to 10% and weight lost will be regained with in a week or two.
   B. Procedure for weight assessment in the newborn.
7. Sensory capabilities of newborn related to sight and sound (pp. 572–573):
   A. Sensory capabilities.
   B. Stimuli parents can provide to foster development.
8. ACROSS; **1.** suck, **2.** habituation, **5.** red, **7.** suture, **9.** milia, **11.** extrusion, **12.** rugae, **13.** one, **14.** colic, **16.** brick, **19.** jaundice, **22.** mongolian spots, **23.** harlequin, **25.** gluteal, **28.** two, **29.** vernix caseosa, **30.** LGA, **31.** SGA, **33.** tonic neck, **34.** tremor, **38.** grasp, **39.** ovale, **40.** smegma, **43.** brown fat, **45.** surfactant, **46.** convection, **49.** evaporation, **50.** peeling, **51.** reflexes.
   DOWN: **1.** strabismus, **3.** three, **4.** moro, **6.** flare, **8.** murmur, **9.** meconium, **10.** acrocyanosis, **15.** lanugo, **17.** hydrocele, **18.** telangiectatic, **20.** cephalhematoma, **21.** pearl, **24.** babinski, **26.** molding, **27.** petechiae, **32.** rooting, **35.** AGA, **36.** apgar, **37.** reactivity, **41.** conduction, **42.** gastrocolic, **44.** toxicum, **47.** creases, **48.** pad.

CHAPTER 21

1. Apgar Scoring: Chapter 18, Fig. 18–4 (p. 492). Baby boy Smith: Score 9 (one point for color due to acrocyanosis), routine supportive care.
   Baby girl Doe: Score 5 (2, 1, 1, 1, 0), respiratory support (pp. 588–592), close observation in protective environment, reduce stressors, and maintain temperature (p. 587).
2. Examination of a 24-hour-old neonate:
   A. Nursing measures to ensure safety, accuracy during the examination (p. 582).
   B. Major points to assess (p. 582).
   C. Parental presence during the examination: answers may vary but should include such factors as increasing parental knowledge of newborn characteristics and behavior (both adaptive and ineffective), providing time to observe parent-newborn interaction, answering

questions, and preparing parents for discharge (pp. 582, 608).

3. Measures to prevent cold stress and overheating:
   —Definitions of each heat transfer mechanism, Chapter 20 (p. 533).
   —Answer should include such areas as temperature considerations during the physical examination (p. 582), measures to maintain body temperature (pp. 587–588), clothing to use (p. 593), and temperature considerations during hygienic care (p. 594).
4. Patent airway
   A. Use of bulb syringe (p. 589).
   B. Use of mechanical suction (p. 590).
5. Measures to alert a drowsy baby: Table 21–1 (p. 583).
6. Assessment and care of the umbilical cord (pp. 593, 596), and new circumcision (p. 604) by parent after discharge.
7. Safety/aseptic principles during the sponge bath: answer should reflect understanding of the concept of medical asepsis as well as awareness of developmental characteristics (pp. 594, 595; Fig. 21–8 [pp. 596, 597]).
8. Hyperbilirubinemia
   A. Response to parental concern regarding jaundice in newborn: answer should reflect basis of elevated bilirubin levels in the newborn using terms parents can understand, with emphasis placed on the normalcy of the occurrence (p. 599, teaching box [p. 601]).
   B. Precautions/care with phototherapy (pp. 599, 602).
9. Importance of immunizations and comparison of immunity received from immunization and from breast-feeding (pp. 610–611).
10. F (p. 587); F (p. 582); T (p. 591); F (p. 589, Fig. 21–2, p. 592)); T (p. 595); T (p. 599); F (p. 604); T (p. 606); F (p. 606); F (p. 608); T (p. 608); F (p. 610).

CHAPTER 22

1. Compute daily calorie/fluid requirements (p. 622): Jim: 417 calories, 405 mL
   Sue: 649–650 calories, 632 mL
   Sam: 718 calories, 770 mL
2. Introduction of solid foods: answers should include readiness (pp. 620–621) and the principles that should be followed (pp. 646–647).
3. Fat requirement of the infant (p. 622).
4. *LACTATION STRUCTURES OF THE BREAST:*
   Fig. 22–2 (p. 624) A. alveolus, **B.** ductule, **C.** duct, **D.** lactiferous duct, **E.** lactiferous sinus, **F.** nipple pore, **G.** ampulla, **H.** areola.
   MILK PRODUCTION REFLEX: Fig. 22–3, *A* (p. 625)
   A. sucking stimulus, **B.** hypothalamus, **C.** anterior pituitary (prolactin), **D.** milk production.
   LET-DOWN REFLEX: Fig. 22–3, *B* (p. 625)
   A. sucking stimulus, **B.** hypothalamus, **C.** posterior pituitary (oxytocin), **D.** let-down.
5. Decision-making related to feeding method:
   A. Couple making the decision together: answer should emphasize the need to parent together and the need to support each other when providing nourishment for their baby especially if breast-feeding is the choice (p. 621).
   B. Making decision prenatally: answer must include need to make the decision in an unrushed manner with time to fully consider the choices (p. 621).
   C. Informed decision-making requires information regarding pros and cons of breast-feeding (p. 628) and bottle-feeding (p. 640) as well as the process of feeding and care required.
6. Breast-feeding:
   A. Let-down (p. 625).
   B. Signs of good nutrition (p. 631).
   C. Sore nipples (p. 630, Table 22–2 [p. 638]).
   D. Engorgement (Table 22–2 [p. 638]).
   E. Afterpains/increased flow (Fig. 22–3, *B* [p. 625], Table 22–2 [p. 639]).
   F. Birth control (p. 637).
7. **A.** (p. 630), **B.** + (p. 630), **C.** + (p. 630), **D.** − (p. 629), **E.** + (p. 629), **F.** − (p. 630), **G.** + (p. 630), **H.** − (p. 637), **I.** − (p. 645).
8. Bottle-feeding:
   A. Maternal concern regarding effect of decision on the baby: answer must emphasize nonjudgmental support of the decision as well as measures the client can use to foster closeness with the newborn and good nutrition (pp. 640, 643).
   B. principles of feeding: feeding skills (p. 641), formula feeding teaching box (p. 643), and formula preparation box (p. 645).

CHAPTER 23

1. Questions/concerns of postpartum woman:
   A. Uterine cramping associated with breast-feeding (p. 658).
   B. Length of time uterine fundus can be palpated through abdomen (p. 658).
   C. Pattern and duration of lochial flow (pp. 659, 660).
   D. Protruding abdomen after birth (p. 661).
   E. Diaphoresis/diuresis: answer should include basis for the occurrence as well as assessment measures being used to rule out infection (p. 666).
2. F (p. 658, Fig. 23–1 [p. 659]), T (p. 658), T (p. 658), F (p. 659), T (p. 660), T (p. 660), F (p. 662), F (pp. 662–663), T (Table 23–3 [p. 664]), F (p. 664), F (p. 665), T (p. 666).
3. ACROSS: **1.** oxytocin, **3.** taking hold, **8.** synchrony, **9.** letting go, **10.** homans sign, **14.** entrainment, **16.** episiotomy, **18.** alba, **19.** serosa, **20.** syometrial, **23.** claiming, **24.** afterpains, **26.** subinvolution **27.** prolactin, **28.** diaphoresis, **29.** taking in, **30.** engorgement.
   DOWN: **2.** orthostatic, **4.** involution, **5.** diastasis recti abdominis, **6.** attachment, **7.** biorhythmicity, **11.** diuresis, **12.** fleshy, **13.** reciprocity, **15.** hemorrhoid, **17.** perperium, **21.** engrossment, **22.** exfoliation, **25.** rubra.

CHAPTER 24

1. Techniques to communicate with a newborn and the manner in which they communicate: touch, eye contact, voice, entrainment, biorhythmicity, reciprocity, and synchrony (pp. 674–677); rhythm, repertoires, responsivity (pp. 683–684); signaling and executive behaviors (p. 673).
2. Maternal concern regarding lack of immediate, early contact with her newborn: answer must reflect a realistic view of early contact that is supported by research findings and reality (pp. 676–677).
3. Parental disappointment in sex and appearance of newborn, reconciling actual child with dream child:
   - Foster attachment/claiming and acquaint parents with their newborn (pp. 673–674).
   - Measures to facilitate their ability to reconcile the actual with the dream child including explanation of appearance and opportunity for parents to discuss their feelings without fear of judgment by the nurse (pp. 678–680).
4. Realistic preparation for and expectations of a three-year-old's adjustment to a newborn sibling (pp. 686–687, Fig. 24–10 and 11 [pp. 688, 689]).
5. Typical behaviors and appropriate nursing measures for each phase of maternal adjustment to the role of parent: taking in (p. 680), taking hold (p. 680–681), and letting go (p. 681).

CHAPTER 25

1. Use of cultural "heat and cold practices" as they relate to food, lactation, ADL, and psychosocial adaptation (pp. 697–699, 716)
2. Elevated temperature 8 hours postpartum following an 18-hour labor:
   - **A.** Assess client for signs and symptoms of infection (p. 700), box—signs of potential physiologic problems, (p. 701).
   - **B.** Dehydration (p. 700).
3. Assessment of episiotomy: answer should include data gathering concerning childbirth events, position, gloves, lighting as well as assessment using the REEDA guidelines (p. 701).
4. Fulfilling request for pain medication: priority approach must be to obtain a full description of the pain being experienced by the client as a guide for appropriate intervention (pp. 706–708).
5. Identification of nursing diagnoses, goals, and interventions: nursing diagnoses and goal statements must reflect current professional guidelines.
   - **A.** High risk for infection of episiotomy related to ineffective perineal self-care practices (pp. 704–706, care box [p. 707]).
   - **B.** Pain related to episiotomy and hemorrhoids (pp. 704–708, care box [p. 707]).
   - **C.** Alteration in bowel elimination: constipation related to inactivity and lack of knowledge regarding measures to promote elimination (p. 711).
   - **D.** Situational low self-esteem related to perceived failure concerning performance during childbirth: integration of the birth experience (pp. 717–718).
   - **E.** Altered parenting related to lack of knowledge and experience concerning infant care measures: transition to the parental role (pp. 718–720).
   - **F.** Ineffective individual coping related to impact of physical and psychosocial changes following childbirth: family adjustment and crisis prevention (p. 720); coping mechanisms (p. 724).
6. D (Table 25–3, p. 705); A (Table 25–3, p. 704); F (Table 25–3, p. 705); E (p. 712); B (p. 707).
7. Health teaching required following administration of rubella immunization (p. 712).
8. Nursing measures related to physician's order "RhoGam if indicated": answer should include confirmation of Rh status of mother and newborn as well as administration guidelines (p. 712).
9. Parental concern regarding their crying infant (pp. 720–721; infant massage box [pp. 722–723]).
10. Alteration in sexuality following childbirth: maternal self-image and sexual adjustment (p. 716), discharge planning (p. 726), box: resumption of sexual intercourse (p. 726) and postbirth contraception (p. 727).

CHAPTER 26

1. Early discharge:
   - **A.** Factors implicated in trend (pp. 736–737).
   - **B.** Advantages (p. 737) and disadvantages (pp. 737–739, Table 26–1 [p. 738]) cited for an early discharge approach.
   - **C.** Counseling a client facing a decision concerning her participation in an early discharge program: assess client and family according to criteria related to early discharge (p. 736), assess level of knowledge concerning early discharge, provide information concerning advantage and disadvantages as they apply to her situation (p. 737–739), include partner in decision making, and provide preparatory classes (pp. 741–743).
2. Early discharge learning needs:
   - **A.** Constraints/barriers to providing required health teaching (pp. 741–742).
   - **B.** Answers may vary, thus providing a good topic for group discussion to consider creative approaches to overcome the constraints/barriers (teaching plan (pp. 742–743); self-assessment of learning needs (table 26–2, p. 744).
3. Advantages and disadvantages for: home visits (pp. 745–753), telephone follow-up (p. 753–756), warm lines (p. 756), support groups (pp. 756–758), and perinatal coaching (pp. 758–759).

CHAPTER 27

1. F (p. 774), T (p. 774), T (p. 775), F (p. 775), T (p. 776), F (p. 776), T (pp. 785, 786), F (p. 788), F (p. 789), F (p. 794), T (pp. 792, 795), F (p. 800).
2. Risk factors for pregnant woman and fetus/neonate at each stage of the childbearing cycle (Table 27–2 [pp. 777–778]; box: factors that place postpartum woman and neonate at high risk [p. 783]).

3. Psychosocial perinatal warning indicators for families at risk for ineffective parenting (Table 27–3 [pp. 779–781]).
4. Preparing pregnant woman and her family for antepartal testing: answers may vary but should reflect use of the nursing process and recognition of family anxiety, lack of knowledge and concerns. This question is ideal for group discussion and could include data from student interviews of clients who have experienced such tests (p. 802).
5. Biophysical profile:
   A. Explanation of the test and its purpose to concerned client (pp. 789–790).
   B. Interpretation of score of 8: factors evaluated and meaning of the score (p. 789, Table 27–7 [p. 790]).
6. C (p. 785–786), E (p. 793), A (p. 789), H (p. 788), I (p. 796), B (pp. 791–792), D (p. 794), J (p. 798), F (p. 795), G (p. 801).
7. Non-stress test:
   A. Client preparation (p. 798).
   B. Protocol to follow in conducting the test (p. 800).
   C. Interpretation of findings: reactive (criteria [p. 800], Table 27–10 [p. 801]); 2. nonreactive (criteria [p. 801], Table 27–10 [p. 801]).
8. Contraction stress test using nipple stimulation:
   A. Client preparation (pp. 801–802).
   B. Protocol to follow in conducting the test (p. 802).
   C. Interpretation of findings: 1. negative (criteria [p. 802], Table 27–11 [p. 803]); 2. positive (criteria [p. 802], Table 27–11 [p. 803]).
9. Nurse's role in the preparation/teaching of client undergoing amniocentesis (pp. 792–794). NOTE: Student may need assistance in delineating the nurse's role.
10. Approach used to determine reproductive health hazards: answer must reflect a holistic approach that includes the environment, the client and her partner, and social and emotional forces (pp. 802–805).

CHAPTER 28

1. Distinguishing factors of hypertensive states associated with pregnancy (pp. 814–815).
2. Expected physiologic adaptations to pregnancy (pp. 815–816; box: changes in normal pregnancy [p. 816]) contrasted with ineffective responses of PIH (pp. 816–820, Fig. 28–1 [p. 818]).
3. D (p. 815), C (p. 815), B (p. 814), E (p. 820), A (p. 815).
4. Mild preeclampsia—home care:
   A. Typical clinical findings (Table 28–1, p. 822).
   B. Organization of home care routine (pp. 828–830).
   C. Health teaching required regarding client/family recognition of health status and signs of advancing PIH (pp. 828–830).
   D. Basis, assessment, prevention of potential complications: pathophysiology (pp. 819–820), assessment measures (pp. 821–827), and prevention measures (pp. 827–830).
5. Severe preeclampsia—hospital care
   A. Typical clinical findings (Table 28–1, p. 822).
   B. Nursing assessment and interventions (pp. 830, 833, 837, 838, 839).
   C. Therapeutic effect of magnesium sulfate (pp. 837, 838).
   D. Assessment measures to detect signs of magnesium toxicity (p. 838).
   E. Antidote for magnesium sulfate: calcium gluconate; drug card should be included (p. 838).

CHAPTER 29

1. Vulnerability to infection during pregnancy:
   A. Rationale (pp. 848, 863).
   B. Preventive measures: answer should reflect understanding of common infections and their mode of transmission (pp. 856, Table 29–1 [p. 857], p. 863; boxes: safer sex; genital hygiene, pp. 869, 873, 876).
2. Self-assessment for the signs/symptoms of genitourinary infections (pp. 863, 866–869) and prevention measures (pp. 863, 869).
3. Chart (mode of transmission, maternal, fetal/neonatal effects, treatment) related to selected infections that can affect the outcome of pregnancy: chlamydia (pp. 848–849), gonorrhea (pp. 849–850), syphilis (pp. 850–853), HPV (p. 859–861), bacterial vaginosis (p. 866), vulvovaginal candidiasis (pp. 866–867), Group B Streptococci (p. 867), pyelonephritis (p. 868), Varicella (p. 874).
4. TORCH infections:
   A. hepatitis A/infectious hepatitis (p. 857), **B.** rubella (p. 857), **C.** toxoplasmosis (p. 855), **D.** cytomegalovirus (p. 857), **E.** hepatitis B/serum hepatitis (p. 857), **F.** herpes simplex virus (p. 857–859).
5. F (p. 848), T (p. 848), T (p. 849), T (pp. 849, 850), F (p. 850), T (p. 851), F (p. 851), T (p. 853), F (p. 855), T (p. 855), F (p. 855).
6. Three principle manifestations of toxic shock syndrome (p. 875).
7. HIV Infection:
   A. Holistic assessment to indicate HIV risk and status (pp. 853–854).
   B. Modes of transmission: mother to fetus/newborn (p. 853).
   C. Nursing measures to support the immune system (pp. 854, 855) and prevent transmission (pp. 855, 877–878).
8. Puerperal infection:
   A. Predisposing factors (p. 870).
   B. Prevention measures (p. 871).
   C. Typical clinical manifestations (pp. 870–871).
   D. Critical treatment measures (p. 871).
   E. Potential sequelae (p. 870).
9. Mastitis: typical manifestations, prevention measures and required treatment/health teaching (pp. 872–873).

CHAPTER 30

1. Threatened abortion:
   A. Basis for signs and symptoms presented (p. 886, Table 30–1 [p. 887]).
   B. Management: answer should reflect a holistic approach that includes not only physical care but also strategies/support measures to meet emotional needs (Table 30–2 [p. 889], p. 890, discharge teaching box [p. 891]).

2. Client reports "good amount of bleeding":
A. Questions asked should reflect knowledge of typical manifestations of spontaneous abortions (Table 30–1 [p. 887], pp. 887–889, box: assessment of bleeding in pregnancy {p. 889}).
B. Incomplete abortion: priority nursing diagnosis must reflect moderate to heavy bleeding: fluid volume deficit related to blood loss associated with spontaneous abortion (pp. 887, 890).
C. Typical nursing interventions (Table 30–2 [p. 889], p. 890).
D. Post-discharge instructions (p. 891).

3. Acute ruptured ectopic pregnancy:
A. Clinical findings (pp. 893, 894–895).
B. Priority nursing diagnosis: decreased cardiac output or fluid volume deficit (p. 895).
C. Nursing care approach (pp. 893–894, 895).

4. Hydatidiform mole: typical clinical manifestations (p. 896–897) and follow-up management (pp. 897–898).

5. Comparison of clinical picture and treatment of marginal placenta previa and abruptio placenta:
A. Clinical picture (pp. 899–901, Table 30–4 [p. 900], pp. 905–906).
B. Nursing care measures (pp. 901, 902, 906–907).
C. Top priorities following birth (pp. 901, 906).

6. E (p. 893), H (p. 886), G (p. 898), A (p. 890), C (p. 895), B (p. 902), D (p. 907), F (p. 912).

7. Postbirth hemorrhage:
A. Contrast causative/risk factors for immediate postbirth hemorrhage with those for delayed postbirth hemorrhage (p. 908).
B. Nursing measures for prevention and early detection (pp. 910—911, 912—913).

8. Mild hemorrhagic shock:
A. Typical manifestations (Table 35, p. 914).
B. Immediate interventions: answer must include recognition of physiologic and emotional needs of the client (pp. 914–917).
C. Ongoing assessment to determine status and response to treatment (pp. 914–917).

9. DIC: predisposing conditions, pathophysiology, clinical manifestations and priority nursing interventions (pp. 917–918).

CHAPTER 31

1. Signs/symptoms with physiologic basis for diabetes mellitus (pp. 924–925).

2. **A.** 5 (p. 924), **B.** carbohydrate, protein, fat, hyperglycemia, insulin, insulin (p. 924), **C.** insulin-dependent, non–insulin-dependent, maturity onset (p. 925), **D.** glycemic control (p. 925), **E.** pregestational diabetes, gestational diabetes (p. 925), **F.** hypoglycemia (p.927), hyperglycemia (p. 927), ketoacidosis (p. 929), **G.** phosphatidylglycerol (pg), L/S ratio (p. 933).

3. Metabolic changes in pregnancy (pp. 925–927) with impact on diabetes (pp. 927–928).

4. Importance of preconception counseling (p. 928).

5. Major maternal and fetal/neonatal risks/complications imposed by pregestational diabetes, their basis and possible prevention measures (pp. 928–931).

6. Type I diabetic—pregnant:
A. Maternal fetal assessment measures required (pp. 931–933).
B. Potential stressors facing the client/family (p. 934).
C. Focus/intervention related to selected factors at each stage of pregnancy: diet (pp. 934, 935, 940), glucose monitoring (pp. 935, 936, 940), insulin requirements (p. 938–939, 940), and general care (pp. 939, 940).

7. Gestational diabetes:
A. Clinical picture (p. 941).
B. Risk factors present: Hispanic, > 30 years, obese, family history (mother), previous pregnancy outcome (9 pound 6 ounce girl), 28th week of pregnancy (p. 941).
C. Pathophysiologic basis for condition (pp. 941, 944).
D. Maternal and fetal/neonatal risks/complications (pp. 945–946).
E. Typical nursing assessment (pp. 946–947) and interventions (pp. 947–948).
F. Prognosis for the future: client health and subsequent pregnancy (p. 948).

8. Type II diabetic—pregnant: rationale for using insulin instead of oral hypoglycemic agents (p. 938).

9. Effect of hypothyroidism (p. 954) and hyperthyroidism (pp. 951, 954) on reproductive well-being and pregnancy.

10. Hyperemesis gravidarum:
A. Physiologic/psychologic assessment factors (p. 949).
B. Priority diagnoses: answers may vary but should include effect of this health problem on fluid and electrolytes, fetal status, emotional status, etc. This question would be a good basis for a postclinical conference, especially if students have had or are having the opportunity to care for clients facing this diagnosis (p. 949).
C. Nursing measures (p. 950).

11. PKU: effects on fetal development and their prevention (p. 955).

CHAPTER 32

1. Cardiac disease during pregnancy:
A. Purpose for heparin (p. 965).
B. Instructions regarding use and effects of heparin (p. 965).
C. Symptomatic with increased activity (p. 962).
D. Physical/psychosocial risk factors (pp. 962–963).
E/F. Signs/symptoms of cardiac decompensation (p. 963, box: warning signs—cardiac decompensation [p. 963]).
G. 28th, 32nd, physiologic cardiac stress is greatest at this time (p. 964).
H. Fetal dangers (p. 962).
I. Nursing interventions to prevent decompensation: holistic approach to limit stress (pp. 964–965).
J. Rationale for: emotional support (p. 967), penicillin prophylaxis (p. 970), epidural anesthesia (p. 970), left side-lying position (p. 970), birth position (p. 970), oxytocin use after delivery (p. 970).
K. postbirth risk factors for cardiac decompensation (p. 971).

L. Postpartum measures to reduce cardiac stress (pp. 971–972).
M. Breast-feeding acceptable (p. 972).
N. Discharge planning (p. 972).

2. F (p. 975), T (p. 974), F (p. 975), T (p. 975), F (p. 976), T (p. 977), F (p. 977), T (p. 978), T (p. 979), F (p. 979), T (p. 982), T (p. 983), F (p. 980).
3. Pregnancy—Paraplegic:
   - **A.** Problems faced and effective measures to deal with them (pp. 981–982).
   - **B.** Manner in which birth is accomplished (p. 982).
   - **C.** Postpartum interventions (p. 984).
5. Trauma during pregnancy:
   - **A.** Factors increasing vulnerability to injury (p. 987).
   - **B.** Pregnant woman (32 weeks) falls from two-step ladder:
     - Focus of nursing assessment (p. 987–988).
     - Influence of pregnancy on interpretation of data (pp. 987–988).
     - Discharge instructions (pp. 986–987).

CHAPTER 33

1. Postpartum blues:
   - **A.** Typical behaviors (pp. 996–997)
   - **B.** Predisposing factors/behaviors indicative of progress to postpartum depression (p. 997).
   - **C.** Relevant nursing diagnoses: answers may vary and can include ineffective family coping, impaired home maintenance, high risk for altered parenting, impaired social interaction, situational low self-esteem (pp. 998–999).
   - **D.** Effective nursing measures (p. 1000).
2. Substance abuse during pregnancy:
   - **A.** General biologic/psychosocial effects on pregnancy (p. 1001).
   - **B.** Factors to consider with alcohol (pp. 1001, 1003), cocaine (pp. 1003, 1004), heroin (p. 1004), methamphetamine (p. 1004), marijuana (p. 1005), phencyclidine (p. 1005).
   - **C.** Goal setting/planning: factors to consider (p. 1005).
   - **D.** Nursing intervention during each stage of pregnancy (pp. 1005–1006).
3. F (p. 1008), T (p. 1009), T (p. 1010), F (p. 1010), T (p. 1010), T (p. 996), F (p. 996), T (Table 33–1, p. 1002), T (p. 1004).
4. Factors that lead poor women to delay entry into prenatal care (pp. 1009–1010).

CHAPTER 34

1. Adolescent sexual behavior:
   - **A.** Contributing factors to earlier onset/increased incidence of sexual activity (pp. 1020–1021).
   - **B.** Reasons for avoiding use of contraceptives (p. 1021).
   - **C.** Criteria/content for effective sex education programs: answers should include the trifold approach of decision-making skills, dealing with peer pressure and involvement with parents and community (p. 1022).
   - **D.** Profile of adolescent at high risk for pregnancy (p. 1023).
2. Impact of adolescence on meeting developmental tasks of pregnancy: accepting reality of pregnancy, unborn child, and parenthood (p. 1023).
3. 16-year-old unwed mother of one-week-old newborn:
   - **A.** Factors that can interfere with an adolescent's ability to meet the tasks of parenthood (p. 1025).
   - **B.** Nursing measures effective in establishing a trusting relationship with adolescent parents (pp. 1036–1038).
4. Consequences of adolescent pregnancy for mother and fetus/newborn both physiologic and socioeconomic (p. 1026). Two-fold role of the nurse aimed at reducing the negative consequences: encourage early, continued prenatal care, and refer to appropriate social support services (p. 1027).
5. 16-year-old sexually active adolescent woman:
   - **A.** Establishing trust and rapport: answer must include recognition of the importance of communication techniques and the environment as well as the sensitivity of this assessment for the adolescent (p. 1027).
   - **B.** Data to be obtained (pp. 1027–1028).
   - **C.** Two priority diagnoses: knowledge deficit related to sexually transmitted diseases and high risk for pregnancy related to sexual activity without contraceptive use (p. 1028).
   - **D.** Interventions (p. 1028).
6. 15-year-old newly diagnosed pregnant woman:
   - **A.** Points to emphasize when assessing an adolescent pregnant woman: answer must be a holistic approach that focuses not only on physiologic factors but also on her reaction and that of her support system to the pregnancy (pp. 1029–1030).
   - **B.** Nursing measures to assist the client to cope with pregnancy and make decisions concerning the future (pp. 1030–1031).
   - **C.** Nursing approaches/interventions at each stage: prenatal (pp. 1031–1033), labor (p. 1034), postpartum (pp. 1034–1036); the developmental needs and concerns of the young adolescent must be considered as part of the answer.

CHAPTER 35

1. Define: **A.** dystocia (p. 1046), **B.** dysfunctional labor (p. 1046), **C.** precipitous labor (p. 1047), **D.** pelvic and soft-tissue dystocia (p. 1047), **E.** cephalopelvic disproportion (p. 1048), **F.** fetal malposition and presentation (p. 1049), **G.** prolonged latent phase (p. 1053), **H.** protracted active phase (p. 1053), **I.** arrested active phase (p. 1053), **J.** protracted descent (p. 1053), **K.** arrested descent (p. 1053), **L.** failure of descent (p. 1053), **M.** external cephalic version (p. 1055), **N.** trial of labor (p. 1055), **O.** induction of labor (p. 1055), **P.** augmentation of labor (p. 1057), **Q.** amniotomy (p. 1056), **R.** forceps-assisted birth (p. 1058), **S.** vacuum extraction (p. 1059), **T.** VBAC (p. 1066).
2. Five factors that lead to dystocia and their interrelationship: dysfunctional labor (pp. 1046–1047), altered pelvic structures (p. 1047), fetal causes (pp. 1047–1051), position of the mother (p. 1051) and psychologic response to labor (pp. 1051–1052).

3. Compare/contrast hypertonic (p. 1046) and hypotonic (p. 1047) labor as to precipitating factors, clinical picture and management. (Table 35–1, p. 1048).
4. LOP with difficulty pushing: nursing measures to assist (pp. 1047, 1051; Fig. 35–2 [p. 1049]).
5. Breech malpresentation: considerations for care (pp. 1049–1051).
6. Induction of labor:
   A. Purpose/criteria for Bishop's score (Table 35–3, p. 1056).
   B. Interpretation of score of "8": favorable score indicating the cervix is ripe/inducible (p. 1056).
   C. Nursing responsibilities with amniotomy: a holistic approach (p. 1056, care box [p. 1059]).
   D. Appropriate actions (pp. 1055–1057, procedure box [p. 1059], 1, 2, 5, 6, 7, 9).
   E. Major side effects: answer should include maternal and fetal side effects along with defining criteria (p. 1057, box: uterine hyperstimulation [p. 1058]).
7. Emergency cesarean birth: good focus for postclinical conference since most students will have had clinical experience with a client who has had a cesarean birth and thus can discuss their approach to care:
   A. Recovery room assessment (pp. 1064–1065).
   B. Appropriate nursing diagnoses: a variety of answers are acceptable but should reflect a holistic focus that takes into consideration not only the client's physiologic needs but also the unexpected nature of the event, and the client's feelings about and perception of the event (pp. 1053–1054).
   C. Nursing interventions (pp. 1064–1066).
8. Preterm labor:
   A. 20th, 37th, PROM, multifetal gestation, hydramnios, incompetent cervix, premature separation of placenta, certain types of infections, unknown, 2/3 (p. 1070), tocolytic (p. 1074), propranolol/inderal (p. 1075), calcium gluconate (p. 1076), betamethasone, 24–48 (p. 1076).
   B. Profile of woman at risk (pp. 1070–1071, box: risk factors for preterm labor [p. 1071]).
   C. Prevention measures: answer should be based upon the known risk factors (pp. 1070–1071, 1074).
   D. Signs of preterm labor to teach a pregnant woman (p. 1073, box: home management of preterm labor, [p. 1074], Chapter 13 [pp. 329–330]).
   E. Actions to take if signs of preterm labor are noted (p. 1073).
   F. Objective signs of preterm labor (p. 1073, 1074, and Chapter 13 [pp. 329–330]).
   G. Nursing measures with clients receiving ritodrine (p. 1074), terbutaline (pp. 1074–1076), and magnesium sulfate (p. 1076).
9. Postterm birth: birth beyond week 42 of gestation: maternal and fetal/neonatal risks (p. 1078).

CHAPTER 36

1. Transitional care nursery:
   A. Progressive signs of neonatal respiratory distress (pp. 1088–1089, Fig. 36–2 [p. 1091]).
   B. Supportive nursing measures to prevent respiratory distress: positioning, suction/patent airway, thermoneutral environment (p. 1092).
2. Oxygen therapy:
   A. Criteria for use (p. 1094).
   B. Purpose/methodology for pulse oximetry (pp. 1094–1095).
   C. Indications and nursing care measures for oxygen administration: hood (p. 1095), continuous positive airway pressure (p. 1096), and mechanical ventilation (pp. 1096–1097).
3. Cold stress:
   A. Signs indicative of cold stress (p. 1098).
   B. Attachment sites for thermistor probe: over the liver and between the umbilicus and the pubis (pp. 1098–1099).
   C. Nursing measures to prevent/minimize cold stress (p. 1099).
4. Preterm newborn: nutritional needs and care
   A. Findings to document following a feeding (pp. 1100–1101).
   B. Weight loss limit in first 3 days: up to 12% of birth weight (p. 1101).
   C. Insertion of gavage tube (p. 1103 and Fig. 36–8).
   D. Principles to guide care before, during, and after a gavage feeding (pp. 1103–1104, p. 1105), non-nutritive sucking.
5. Intensive care nursery:
   A. Infant stressor (pp. 1107–1108) and family stressors (pp. 1111, 1112), including anticipatory grief.
   B. Cues for neonatal overstimulation and measures to limit stimuli (p. 1108) and signs of readiness for interaction and measures to provide sensory stimulation (p. 1108 and 1109), kangaroo care.

CHAPTER 37

1. Terminology related to gestational age and birth weight (p. 1120): **A.** preterm/premature, **B.** term, **C.** postterm, **D.** postmature, **E.** large for gestational age (LGA), **F.** appropriate for gestational age (AGA), **G.** small for gestational age (SGA), **H.** intrauterine growth retardation (IUGR), **I.** low birth weight (LBW), less than expected rate of intrauterine growth, shortened gestational period, **J.** 2500 g (5 1/2 pounds), 37 weeks.
2. Gestational age assessment (pp. 1121–1127): P, T, P, P, P, P, T, T, P, T, P, T, P.
3. Vulnerability of preterm infant related to maintenance of body temperature (p. 1128), respiratory function (p. 1128), nutritional/glucose balance (p. 1128), resistance to infection (p. 1128), maintenance of renal function (p. 1128), hematologic status (p. 1128), responsiveness to parents (p. 1130).
4. Parental responses to preterm newborn:
   A. Stages of response (pp. 1129, 1130); B, C, A, B, A, C.
   B. Nursing support measures (p. 1134).
5. Prolonged pregnancy:
   A. Assessment findings suggestive of prolonged pregnancy and postmaturity (p. 1140).
   B. Dangers facing postmature, LGA fetus/newborn during labor, birth, and the postbirth periods (pp. 1143–1144).

6. Four major complications faced by SGA/IUGR fetus/newborn: perinatal asphyxia, meconium aspiration, hypoglycemia, heat loss (p. 1142).

CHAPTER 38

1. Hyperbilirubinemia:
   A. Differentiate physiologic (pp. 1151, 1152–1153, 1154–1155) from pathologic (pp. 1150–1151, 1151–1152, 1154–1155) hyperbilirubinemia as to onset, causes, and treatment.
   B. Jaundice (icterus) (p. 1150); kernicterus (p. 1150).
   C. Physiology of hyperbilirubinemia (p. 1152).
   D. Preventive measures (p. 1154).
   E. Nursing measures: nursing measures for phototherapy: case study/care plan (pp. 1155–1156), Chapter 22.
2. Rh-negative woman–second pregnancy:
   A. Indirect Coombs' positive: meaning (p. 1151).
   B. Not a candidate for RhoGAM (pp. 1151, 1154).
   C. Use of RhoGAM (p. 1154).
   D. Erythroblastosis fetalis (pp. 1150, 1152).
3. Congenital disorders:
   A. Meaning of congenital and genetic (p. 1156).
   B. Multisystem signs indicative of congenital disorders: neurologic (p. 1158), cardiovascular (p. 1158), respiratory (p. 1157), gastrointestinal (p. 1158), urogenital (p. 1159), musculoskeletal (p. 1158), Table 38–1 [p. 1161]).
4. Briefly describe: inborn errors of metabolism (p. 1162), diaphragmatic hernia (p. 1164), tracheoesophageal fistula (p.1165), esophageal atresia (p. 1165), omphalocele (p. 1165), imperforate anus (p. 1166), congenital hip dysplasia (p. 1168), exstrophy of the bladder (p. 1170), epispadias (p. 1171), hydrocephalus (p. 1168), anencephaly (p. 1168), microcephaly (p. 1168), meningomyelocele (p. 1167), meningocele (p. 1167), talipes equinovarus (p. 1170), polydactyly (p. 1170), hypospadias (p. 1171), ambiguous genitalia (p. 1171).
5. Supportive care for parents: newborn with cleft lip and palate (pp. 1168–1169, pp. 1172–1173).

CHAPTER 39

1. Birth injuries:
   A. Risk factors related to mother, fetus, and intrapartum events/birth techniques (p. 1180).
   B. Signs of fractured clavicle (p. 1182).
2. T (p. 1180), T (p. 1181), F (p. 1181), T (p. 1182), F (p. 1182), T (p. 1185), F (p. 1195), F (p. 1196), T (p. 1198), T (p. 1198), T (p. 1198), F (p. 1199), T (p. 1199), T (p. 1205), F (p. 1207), T (p. 1209).
3. Decrease, 2 to 6 times more common, blood glucose levels, ketoacidosis, hyperglycemia, glucose, insulin, growth, macrosomia, acidic, carbon dioxide, oxygen, glucose (p. 1185), 100–200, 300, glycosuria, ketonuria, ketoacidosis (p. 1188).
4. Macrosomic newborn of pregestational diabetic mother: typical characteristics and signs of complications (pp. 1186–1188).
5. Infection—fetus/newborn:
   A. Modes of transmission throughout pregnancy (p. 1191).
   B. Risk factors for neonatal infection (p. 1192).
   C. Signs indicative of infection (pp .1192–1193).
   D. Nursing measures related to prevention, cure, rehabilitation (pp. 1194–1195).
6. Infant of HBV-positive mother: protocol to follow with infant (p. 1196).
7. Active genital herpes at vaginal birth:
   A. Four modes of transmission to newborn (p. 1194).
   B. Clinical signs of active newborn infection (p. 1200).
   C. Nursing measures related to parental teaching, health care follow up for infant, and vidarabine/acyclovir therapy (p. 1200–1201).
8. Infant or HIV-positive mother:
   A. Potential for newborn infection (p. 1201).
   B. Positive, 8–15 months (p. 1202).
   C. Two diagnostic infections: lymphoid interstitial pneumonitis and recurrent oral candidiasis (p. 1202).
   D. HIV present in breast milk (p. 1201); therefore should not breast-feed (p. 1202).
9. Thrush:
   A. Signs exhibited by newborn (p. 1203).
   B. Mode of transmission (p. 1203).
   C. Nursing interventions (p. 1203).
10. Fetal alcohol syndrome (FAS):
   A. Characteristics exhibited (pp. 1205–1206).
   B. Nursing diagnoses related to altered thought process and perception as well as intellectual and communication deficits (p. 1207).
   C. Nursing measures to facilitate growth and development (p. 1207).
11. Maternal substance abuse during pregnancy and the effect on the fetus/newborn:
   A. Clinical withdrawal picture for heroin (pp. 1207, 1209), methadone (p. 1209) and cocaine (p. 1209–1210).
   B. General nursing care measures (pp. 1203–1205).

CHAPTER 40

1. Dimensions of mourning (pp. 1218–1219):
   A. shock and numbness,
   B. searching and yearning,
   C. disorganization,
   D. reorganization.
2. Worden's four tasks of mourners (pp. 1219–1220).
3. Aftermath of a spontaneous abortion at 10 weeks' gestation:
   A. Approach for individualized care: answer must focus on the compassionate gathering of information regarding the meaning of this pregnancy and the impact of its loss on the woman and her family in order to obtain a complete picture upon which care will be based (pp. 1221–1222).
   B. Three nursing measures to include in the plan: answers may vary. It would be helpful to use this question as a basis for group discussion to help students work through some of their feelings regarding loss and death especially in terms of pregnancy (pp. 1223–1226).
   C. Therapeutic and nontherapeutic communication and counseling techniques (pp. 1223–1226): N, T, N, N, T, T, N
4. Factors that influence a person's response to loss (p. 1226).
5. Physical needs of a woman experiencing a stillbirth at 38 weeks' gestation (pp. 1226–1227).

6. Viewing of a baby with multiple anomalies: decision-making and measures to make the experience a positive one (p. 1227).
7. Bereavement: distinguishing signs of complicated bereavement and the nursing approach required (pp. 1236–1237).

CHAPTER 41

1. F (p. 1247), T (p. 1247), T (p. 1249), F (Table 41–1, p. 1250), F (p. 1252), F (p. 1252), T (p. 1253), F (p. 1254), F (p. 1256), F (p. 1261), T (p. 1260), F (p. 1262), T (p. 1272).
2. Menstrual disorders:
  A. Factors implicated in hypogonadotrophic amenorrhea (p. 1252).
  B. Nursing diagnoses and relief measures regarding dysmenorrhea: pain related to uterine cramping during the menstrual cycle and knowledge deficit related to relief measures for primary dysmenorrhea (p. 1252).
  C. Effective relief measures for PMS (p. 1253, case study/care plan [pp. 1254–1255]).
  D. Signs/symptoms with pathophysiologic basis for endometriosis (pp. 1254–1256).
  E. Medication cards for danozol and narafelin: evaluate cards for content as outlined and reliability of reference used.
3. Chart (manifestations, physiologic/psychosocial basis, therapeutic measures) related to symptomatology of the climacterium and postclimacterium: vasomotor instability (pp. 1258–1259; 1264), emotional disturbances (pp. 1259–1260), genital atrophy (pp. 1260, 1265), osteoporosis (pp. 1260–1261; 1265–1266), alterations in sexuality (pp. 1262–1263; 1264–1265).
4. Clinical manifestations of cystocele/rectocele (pp. 1267–1269).
5. Osteoporosis:
  A. Risk factors present in the situation given: slender body build, caucasian, sedentary job as secretary, diet low in calcium but high in caffeine and fat, smokes one pack per day, mother had signs of osteoporosis (p. 1261).
  B. Preventive measures (p. 1265, box: prevention of osteoposis [p. 1266]).
6. ACROSS: **3.** endometriosis, **4.** vasomotor, **5.** vesicovaginal, **6.** amenorrhea, **7.** atrophy, **9.** papanicolaou smear, **11.** premenstrual syndrome, **14.** nafarelin, **17.** climacterium, **18.** rectocele, **19.** danozol, **21.** enterocele, **22.** premenopause, **23.** stress incontinence, **24.** osteoporosis.
DOWN: **1.** dysmenorrhea, **2.** retroversion, **4.** vaginal atresia, **8.** prolapse, **9.** perimenopause, **10.** dysplasia, **12.** dyspareunia, **13.** menopause, **15.** postmenopause, **16.** fistula, **17.** cystocele, **20.** pessary.

CHAPTER 42

1. T (p. 1280), F (p. 1280), F (p. 1280), T (pp. 1280, 1281), F (p. 1281), T (p. 1281), F (p. 1283), T (pp. 1286, 1288), F (p. 1289), F (p. 1290), T (p. 1291), T (p. 1293), T (p. 1296), T (p. 1301), F (p. 1308), T (p. 1309), F (p. 1313), F (p. 1313), T (p. 1318), T (p. 1319), T (p. 1328), F (p. 1328).
2. E (Table 42–1, p. 1284), C (p. 1284), B (Table 42–1, p. 1284), D (p. 1285), A (p. 1286).
3. Interrelated structures, functions, and processes essential for conception with emphasis on the couple as a biologic unit (pp. 1281–1282).
4. Diagnostic laparoscopy:
  A. Performed early in the menstrual cycle (p. 1286).
  B. Preoperative care (p. 1286).
  C. Explanation to client regarding what the test encompasses (p. 1286).
  D. Postoperative care measures (p. 1286).
  E. Discharge instructions: answer should include activity precautions, expected discomfort and signs of infection (not in text) (p. 1287).
5. Medication cards for clomiphene, bromocriptine, human menopausal gonadotropin, gonadrotropin-releasing hormone: evaluate each card for content as outlined and reliability of reference used.
6. Testing for impaired fertility—semen analysis:
  A. Procedure (p. 1292).
  B. Box: assessment of the man (p. 1291).
  C. Postcoital test (p. 1292).
  D. Nursing support measures when working with the infertile couple: answer should reflect sensitivity to the emotional impact that infertility and testing required may have on the couple and their relationship (pp 1294–1297).
7. Alternative birth technologies:
  A. Description of in vitro fertilization and embryo transfer (p. 1297), GIFT (p. 1298), zygote intrafallopian transfer (p. 1298), therapeutic intrauterine insemination (p. 1299).
  B. Concerns engendered: answer should include cost as well as physical, emotional, and ethical factors (pp. 1297–1300).
8. Nursing approach to informed decision making regarding contraception: answer should focus on holistic assessment and development of a trusting, therapeutic relationship (pp. 1300–1301).
9. Periodic abstinence methods of contraception:
  A. 8, 21 (p. 1303).
  B. drop, 0.1° F, progesterone, rise, 0.4°-0.8° F, 2-4 days, thermal shift, the day of the drop, 3 days (pp. 1303, 1304).
  C. Cervical mucus, amount, consistency (p. 1304).
  D. BBT, cervical mucus, increased libido, midcycle spotting, mittelschmerz, pelvic fullness/tenderness, vulvar fullness (p. 1305).
  E. LH, 12-24 (pp. 1305–1306).
10. I (p. 1307), C (p. 1307), I (p. 1307), C (p. 1308), I (p. 1308), C (p. 1309), I (p. 1309).
11. Oral contraception—combination estrogen/progestin:
  A. Mode of action (p. 1310).
  B. Absolute and relative contraindications (p. 1311).
  C. Side effects as to estrogen excess (p. 1311), progestin excess (p. 1312), and progestin deficiency (p. 1312).
  D. Meaning of ACHES (p. 1313).
  E. Ensuring maximum effectiveness (p. 1313).
12. Diaphragm use (p. 1314, box: use and care of the diaphragm [pp. 1315–1316]). I, C, C, I, I
13. Cervical cap (pp. 1314, 1317, box: use and care of the cervical cap [p. 1317]).

14. Copper-T 380A IUD: discharge instructions post-IUD insertion (pp. 1318–1319, box: IUD warning signs [p. 1318]).
15. Sterilization:
    A. Nursing approach to decision making with a couple: answer should reflect an unbiased, nonjudgmental approach that includes discussion of feelings, methods, effects (pp. 1319, 1321, 1322).
    B. preoperative and postoperative care related to a vasectomy (pp. 1323–1324).
16. Rights of client and nurse regarding abortion: NAACOG (p. 1325).
17. Decision-making regarding elective abortion:
    A. Nursing approach: answer must reflect an unbiased, nonjudgmental approach that presents the pros and cons of the options available and explore the client's feelings (pp. 1325–1326).
    B. Explanation of laminaria use and uterine aspiration (pp. 1326–1327).
    C. Nursing diagnoses: may vary but should reflect a holistic focus. This would be a good area for a group discussion and exploration of feelings (p. 1326).
    D. Nursing measures related to physical care and emotional support (p. 1327).
    E. Discharge instructions (pp. 1327, 1328).

CHAPTER 43

1. Define: battery (p. 1338), sexual assault (p. 1338), abuse (p. 1338), domestic violence (p. 1340), childhood sexual abuse (p. 1347), childhood sexual assault (p. 1347), incest (p. 1347), rape (p. 1349), acquaintance rape (p. 1350), blitz rape (p. 1350).
2. Supply facts to disprove myths: A, B, C, D, E (p. 1342), F (pp. 1343, 1344).
3. Women as victims of abuse:
    A. Profile of woman most vulnerable (p. 1340, Table 43–1 [p. 1341]).
    B. Four types of men most likely to become abusive husbands: controller, defender, approval seeker, incorporator (pp. 1340–1341).
4. Cyclic nature of battering:
    A. Characteristic behaviors of the three phases: tension building (p. 1341), acute battering incident (p. 1341), and kindness and contrite, loving behavior (p. 1343); Also see Fig. 43–1 (p. 1342).
    B. Implications for anticipatory guidance (pp. 1345–1346).
5. Cues of physical abuse:
    A. Cues (p. 1344).
    B. Process to follow based on suspicion of abuse (p. 1344).
    C. Nursing measures following confirmation by the woman (pp. 1345–1346, box: helper responses—facilitative, [p. 1345]).
    D. Inhibitive responses (box: helper responses—inhibitive [p. 1345]).
    E. Analysis of responses (pp. 1345–1346), the first and the last statements are facilitative responses.
6. Adult survivor of sexual abuse:
    A. Behaviors reflective of delayed onset, posttraumatic stress disorder (pp. 1347–1348).
    B. Effective nursing responses/actions (pp. 1348–1349).
7. Rape:
    A. Collection of evidence (p. 1353).
    B. Meeting of immediate emotional needs (p. 1353, 1354–1355); this question may be used as a basis for classroom discussion of this issue along with exploration of student feelings.
    C. Phases of the rape trauma syndrome (p. 1351); C, A, A, C, B, D, A, A, B, D.

CHAPTER 44

1. C (p. 1374), F (p. 1364, 1365), G (p. 1371), A (p. 1364), B (p. 1371), D (p. 1378), E (p. 1390).
2. T (p. 1364), T (p. 1365), F (p. 1365), F (p. 1371), T (p. 1374), T (p. 1379), F (p. 1380), T (p. 1381), F (p. 1387), T (p. 1391), T (p. 1392), T (p. 1392), F (p. 1393), F (p. 1395), T (p. 1396).
3. Fibrocystic breast disease:
    A. Clinical manifestations (p. 1364).
    B. Suggested relief measure (p. 1364).
4. Breast cancer—modified radical mastectomy:
    A. Risk factors for breast cancer (pp. 1365–1366).
    B. Emotional impact on client and family (p. 1369).
    C. Nursing supportive measures for client and family (p. 1370).
    D. Priority nursing care measures during preoperative (p. 1370), immediate postoperative (p. 1370), and convalescent phases (pp. 1370, 1371, box: postmastectomy arm exercises).
    E. Discharge instructions (p. 1370, box: discharge teaching [p. 1371]).
5. Fibroid tumors:
    A. Clinical manifestations (p. 1372).
    B. Severity of symptoms, age of client, regular checkups, myomectomy, hysterectomy (pp. 1372, 1374).
6. Endometrial cancer:
    A. Nursing care and support measures required during the preoperative (pp. 1375–1376), postoperative (pp. 1376–1377) and convalescent periods (p. 1377).
    B. Discharge instructions (p. 1377, box; the client with a radical hysterectomy [p. 1377]).
7. Risk factors for cervical cancer [pp. 1378–1379].
8. Invasive cervical carcinoma—radiation therapy:
    A. Table related to care before, during, and after internal radiation (pp. 1386–1388) and external radiation (pp. 1385–1386).
    B. Nursing precautions for self-protection during internal radiation therapy (pp. 1386, 1387, Fig. 44–11).
9. Radical Vulvectomy:
    A. Nursing actions related to infection prevention (p. 1390).
    B. Nursing actions related to maintenance of sexual functioning (p. 1390).
    C. Discharge instructions (box: home care of client undergoing radical vulvectomy [p. 1390]).
10. Ovarian cancer: why the "silent disease" (p. 1391).
11. Issues and feelings confronting a pregnant woman, her family, and health care providers when a diagnosis of cancer is made (pp. 1392, 1395, 1396).